Statistics for Laboratory Scientists and Clinicians
A Practical Guide

Understanding the underlying principles of statistical techniques and effectively applying statistical methods can be challenging for researchers at all stages of their career. This concise, practical guide uses a simple, engaging approach to take scientists and clinicians working in laboratory-based life science and medical research through the steps of choosing and implementing appropriate statistical methods to analyze data. The author draws on her extensive experience of advising students and researchers over the past 35 years, breaking down complex concepts into easy-to-understand units. Practical examples using free online statistical tools are included throughout, with illustrations and diagrams employed to keep jargon to a minimum. Sample size calculations and considerations are covered in depth, and the book refers to the types of experiment and data that lab-based scientists are likely to encounter. Straightforward, accessible, and encouraging throughout, this is a go-to reference for researchers who want to achieve statistical autonomy.

Anne McDonnell Sill is a statistician and epidemiologist in the Department of Surgery, Saint Agnes Hospital, Baltimore, MD. She has previously worked as a research associate in the Department of Biostatistics at the Children's National Medical Centre, Washington, D.C., at the Institute of Human Virology (IHV), University of Maryland, Baltimore, MD, and at the Johns Hopkins School of Medicine and School of Hygiene, Baltimore, MD. She has spent more than 35 years advising students, laboratory scientists, and clinicians on experimental design and statistical analysis. She has also used her data management and clinical research experience to help implement public health programs globally, as a consultant for the Centers for Disease Control (CDC).

Statistics for Laboratory Scientists and Clinicians

A Practical Guide

Anne McDonnell Sill
Saint Agnes Hospital, Baltimore, MD

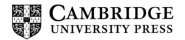

CAMBRIDGE
UNIVERSITY PRESS

University Printing House, Cambridge CB2 8BS, United Kingdom

One Liberty Plaza, 20th Floor, New York, NY 10006, USA

477 Williamstown Road, Port Melbourne, VIC 3207, Australia

314–321, 3rd Floor, Plot 3, Splendor Forum, Jasola District Centre, New Delhi – 110025, India

103 Penang Road, #05-06/07, Visioncrest Commercial, Singapore 238467

Cambridge University Press is part of the University of Cambridge.

It furthers the University's mission by disseminating knowledge in the pursuit of education, learning, and research at the highest international levels of excellence.

www.cambridge.org
Information on this title: www.cambridge.org/9781108477253
DOI: 10.1017/9781108769457

© Anne McDonnell Sill 2021

First published 2021

Printed in the United Kingdom by TJ Books Limited, Padstow Cornwall

A catalogue record for this publication is available from the British Library.

ISBN 978-1-108-47725-3 Hardback
ISBN 978-1-108-70850-0 Paperback

Additional resources for this publication at www.cambridge.org/mcdonnellsill.

Cambridge University Press has no responsibility for the persistence or accuracy
of URLs for external or third-party internet websites referred to in this publication
and does not guarantee that any content on such websites is, or will remain,
accurate or appropriate.

Contents

Preface

This book targets researchers working in laboratory-based life science and medical research areas. The intention is to provide a concise and accessible guide for this audience so that they may understand the underlying principles of these statistical techniques and how to effectively apply these methods in their work. The author's strengths are her extensive experience in helping such individuals with their statistical tasks, and her ability to understand their needs and to communicate effectively with them.

From the author's 35 years of experience in the provision of epidemiological and statistical expertise to a multitude of audiences, her aim was to provide a statistical guide that would appeal to a wide variety of practicing, medical, and laboratory academicians and researchers. Providing links to online statistical tools,* this *practical* and interactive guide will act as a bench-side tool to assist the user in specific areas that are commonly used for interpreting results and preparing or reviewing manuscripts.

Intended key audiences include graduate students who lack the time to revisit their statistics books but need immediate consultation to complete the statistical section of their dissertations, scientists who evaluate a manuscript but fly past the statistical methods section due to their discomfort with statistics, and laboratory scientists who need to know how many specimens to include in an experiment to evaluate the sensitivity and specificity of a test against a gold standard. Readers should benefit from this interactive guide, which will quickly provide solutions to their many statistical inquires. A concise and well-organized guide should address the majority of statistical questions that these groups of professionals will encounter.

Step-by-step considerations are now available in this "how-to" guide. Now with the immediately available and free tools mentioned in this guide, those wanting to conduct such analyses can do so without seeking outside statistical consultation. But, more importantly, and in plain English, this guide will explain how to select the appropriate analytic approach to making sample size or power calculations. Immediately applicable, this guide covers

---

* The full list of links is also available on www.cambridge.org/mcdonnellsill.

the critical examples of the most commonly used techniques used to evaluate data in a simple and effective manner with online assistance.

The Accreditation Council for Graduate Medical Education (ACGME) requires that during their residency programs, physicians must engage in a scholarly activity and produce at least one published article to graduate from the residency program. Toward that goal, residents must often employ statistical techniques with which they may not be familiar. This guide would provide that statistical foundation. For the blood bank laboratorian who screens blood for infectious agents and who must calculate test efficiency, for the cardiologist who must know how many patients to randomize to drug A and drug B to demonstrate drug superiority or equivalency, and to the Institutional Review Board (IRB) reviewer who must evaluate study design and statistical approaches to determine risk and proper statistical methodology, a simple "quick read" of its concisely written sections should provide the reviewer with the confidence to accurately assess the integrity of the research protocol. Some might consider this guide a "necessity," providing as it does an interactive and compact glance at most common statistical tools used in manuscripts, protocols, and scientific inquiry.

As an example, this guide will build upon the technicalities of the normal distribution simply to coach the reader to fully understand their data. Knowing the distributional normality of their data, or lack thereof, guides one to select the appropriate statistical test to analyze that data. Even seasoned scientists have often presented parametric tests on non-normally distributed data such as the $\log_{10}$ HIV viral load, which is a mathematical blunder that could have been avoided had they consulted a guide such as this.

So, at the urging of her colleagues, the author has downloaded her thoughts into this interactive guide so that colleagues can be directed to specific sections of the book, rather than continually having to ask her to calculate their 95% confidence intervals or to "power" their study. The premise of this statistical guide is to explain complex statistical topics in a manner that will not overwhelm or intimidate the medical professional with impenetrable statistical jargon, so that they can immediately apply these methods in their everyday practices.

Acknowledgments

Had it not been for Niel Constantine, PhD (Professor of Pathology, University of Maryland, Baltimore, MD), this book would not have been written. My sincerest thanks go out to Niel for his patience, and his hours upon hours of multiple chapter reviews, edits, comments, and additions, which have brought this book to light. Thank you Dan Edelman, PhD (Head, Clinical Molecular Profiling Core, National Cancer Institute) for your encouragement at the outset of this endeavor. I am also indebted to statisticians Hamid Ferdosi, PhD (George Washington University) and Bilal Khokhar, PhD (Senior Analyst, General Dynamics Health Solutions Contractor) for their statistical reviews and very helpful comments. Thanks also go to Jim Kaper, PhD (Chair, Department of Microbiology & Immunology; Vice Dean for Academic Affairs, University of Maryland, Baltimore, MD) for his first review and endorsement of this book while it was in its concept phase. To my mentors, J. Robert McCarter, ScD (Children's National Medical Center), Farley Cleghorn, MD, MPH (Global Head, Health Practice, Palladium Group), Joann Boughman, PhD (Senior Vice Chancellor for Academic Affairs at the University System of Maryland), Gary Chase, PhD, and Susan Folstein, MD (Johns Hopkins University School of Medicine), I have been honored to be your student and I thank you for your inspiration and your patience as I absorbed your wisdom over so many years. To my parents, Bill and Connie McDonnell, thank you for your love and for your insistence that we "speek and rite" properly as we were growing up, and to my sisters Liz Belli and Kate McDonnell, thank you for your friendship, support, and encouragement. And finally, to my husband, Brian, and my awesome children, Connie and Eddie, thank you for always being the daily mainstay of my being!

I Basic Statistical Concepts

1 Understanding Some Basic Statistical Concepts

1.1 Sample vs. Population

A concept that may not have been well explained in your statistics class of long ago, is sample vs. population estimates. If your mission is to measure weight on all patients with diabetes in the world (or what statisticians call the "universe"), we must measure the **mean** and **standard deviation** (SD) in a representative **sample** of patients that estimates the mean and variance of weight in the **universe** (μ or **standard error**, SE). Thus, we make estimates of population weight through a sample of diabetic patients, for example. By examining samples of data, we are always estimating characteristics of the universe. Ideally, these samples are randomly selected from the population and thus, if we were to choose another random sample from the same population, the results would be approximately equal, within the acceptable bounds of random error. This is why the sample selection becomes critical; the sample must be as representative of the population being studied as possible.

1.2 General Data Management Considerations

If you have a binary variable, i.e., a variable with only two choices, such as gender, in a dataset, it is necessary to always enter the binary code, or leave it blank if it is missing. Too often I have received datasets for analysis that contain a 1 for "yes" and blank for "no," meaning to me that all of the blanks are missing. However, when I asked the author of the dataset about these missing values: "did the patient have cardiovascular disease (CVD)?," she said "oh, no, a blank means that they did not have the CVD." Those missing fields were corrected to receive a value of 0, while the truly missing values were simply left blank. Make no assumptions if you see a lot of missing data.

Another tragic example was when a post-doc decided not to consult the codebook to define who was on study drug and who was on placebo, so he switched the assignments, and in his post-doctoral dissertation, he reported that patients on the study drug did not benefit while the controls did benefit, when indeed the reverse was true. Always document variable codes in a codebook or in the database itself.

Laboratory personnel also need to have access to statisticians, or they should possess a foundational and functional level of knowledge in statistics in order to understand, apply, and interpret their laboratory results and keep their instruments calibrated. Or, they are advised to speak to a statistician at the very start of study development. There can be struggles between laboratory personnel and statisticians/epidemiologists when it comes to data handling or interpretation. As one who helped a lab to optimize the performance of their assays, I would sometimes experience comments like, "oh, we eliminated the outliers," or when data are missing for a certain field, they enter a QNS (quantity not sufficient) instead of leaving it blank, or entering dates as month/day/year in some of the fields and then day/month/year in others, thereby throwing off the date format recognition of my analysis software. So, my best advice is to speak to your statistician before designing your study and your database to discuss:

- study design
- developing the hypothesis and the null hypothesis
- sample size... sample size... sample size... sample size...
- Also, develop a data codebook (including strict formats for dates!).
- Keep ALL data and don't throw out the outliers!

1.3   Central Limit Theorem

Another related concept is the **Central Limit Theorem**, which simply posits that when one continually draws samples from a population and measures their HbA1c levels, for example, the HbA1c values from multiple subjects will eventually take on a normal distribution as one keeps sampling, that is, when plotted the values will take on a bell-shaped distribution that is centered around the mean and the median of the distribution, but only if the values are capable of being normally distributed in the first place. For example, you wouldn't expect a logarithmically distributed variable to eventually take on a normal distribution after repeated sampling because it will always be logarithmically distributed. More on that in Section 2.2.

1.4   Parametric vs. Non-parametric Analyses

We will learn about different types of analyses to perform on different types of data, but the initial question to ask is: "Are the data normally distributed?" If yes, use the parametric statistics toolbox. If they are otherwise, i.e., not normally distributed, use the non-parametric toolbox.

Parametric statistics are a set of statistical procedures that are conducted on normally distributed, continuous variables. Parametric statistics are generally more robust than non-parametric statistics, so it becomes understandable why efforts are often made to "normalize" non-normally distributed data (see Chapter 4) before subjecting them to parametric statistics. For example, HIV viral load must be $\log_{10}$ transformed to assimilate a normal distribution before being analyzed using the parametric T-test.

Non-parametric statistics are a set of statistical procedures that are performed on non-normally distributed data like binary, ordinal, and nominal variables, or on continuous variables that are not normally distributed.

Borrowed and adapted from Tanya Hoskin, a statistician in the Mayo Clinic Department of Health Sciences Research who provides consultations through the Mayo Clinic CTSA BERD Resource,[1] Table 1.1 elucidates which test to use in different circumstances by giving laboratory and clinical examples.

1.5   How to Calculate Some Basic Measures of Central Tendency

The mean, median, and mode are common indices used to describe the characteristics of a sample. They are simple to calculate and give some useful information on how sample values, like age and gender, are distributed; the indices can also be used to compare age and gender between different populations. However, the value of these indices has limitations, and misuse can yield misleading information. Following the definitions and the way to calculate the mean, median, and mode (below), two

Table 1.1   The selection of appropriate statistical tests is dependent on data type

Analysis type	Example	Parametric procedure	Non-parametric procedure
Compare means between two distinct and independent groups	Mean systolic blood pressure for patients on placebo vs. patients on study drug	Two-sample *T*-test	Wilcoxon rank-sum test
Compare two quantitative measurements taken from the same individual	Cell viability before vs. after 3 days in −80F freezer	Paired *T*-test	Wilcoxon signed-rank test
Compare means between three or more distinct/ independent groups	We want to compare the baseline ages of 3 groups: drug #1 vs. drug #2 vs. placebo	Analysis of variance (ANOVA)	Kruskal–Wallis test
Estimate the degree of association between two quantitative values	Viral particles in urine vs. saliva specimens	Pearson correlation	Spearman–Rank correlation

examples of populations are illustrated to make the point of the use and misuse of these measures.

1.5.1   Mean

The **mean** is calculated as the sum of the values divided by the number of the values. Why are means important? Because they give us a single summary value that describes one measure of the data that is useful for comparing across two or more populations.

Calculation of the mean:

What is the mean of 2, 3, 6, and 10?
   Answer: $(2 + 3 + 6 + 10)/4 = 21/4 = 5.25$.

However, if you have a distribution such as the following:
   What is the mean of 20 + 2 + 500 + 2500?

Table 1.2   Frequency distribution of Measured Blood Loss

		Frequency	Percent	Cumulative Percent
		MBL		
Valid	1.50	1	4.3	5.3
	1.54	1	4.3	10.5
	1.64	1	4.3	15.8
	1.78	1	4.3	21.1
	3.55	1	4.3	26.3
	3.70	1	4.3	31.6
	3.78	1	4.3	36.8
	4.27	1	4.3	42.1
	4.93	1	4.3	47.4
	6.41	1	4.3	52.6
	7.21	1	4.3	57.9
	7.39	1	4.3	63.2
	7.53	1	4.3	68.4
	7.84	1	4.3	73.7
	8.02	1	4.3	78.9
	8.63	1	4.3	84.2
	11.28	1	4.3	89.5
	13.43	1	4.3	94.7
	68.83	1	4.3	100.0
	Total	19	82.6	
Missing		4	17.4	
Total		23	100.0	

You might decide that finding the mean of this distribution may be meaningless since there is just so much space between the values. A way to reduce the space is by "normalizing" these values before taking the mean of them (see Section 1.4).

1.5.2   Median

The **median** is the midpoint of a frequency distribution where 50% of values fall below it and 50% of values fall above it. The median can be estimated by constructing a frequency distribution table.

As can be seen from Table 1.2, the midpoint of "Measured Blood Loss" can be found by looking at the cumulative frequency and finding that the

50% mark of the distribution falls somewhere between 4.93 and 6.41. These two values are almost equally distant from 50%, so we can approximate the median by taking the mean of these two values: $(4.93 + 6.41)/2 = 5.67 =$ the median.

1.5.3   Mode

The **mode** is the number that is repeated most frequently in a distribution. If there is a tie between two values, the distribution is said to be bimodal. If three or more values are tied, it is said to be multimodal. Mode can also be used in cases of ordinal variables like race; which race is most prevalent in the ordinal continuum of the race values?

Calculation of the mode:

> What is the mode of 1, 4, 2, 4, 7, 5, 6, 4, 3, 7, 4, 4, 7, 7, and 7?
> **Answer:** 4 and 7. This is a bimodal distribution.

Now, let's examine two different samples and see how the mean, median, and mode represent the samples and their usefulness.

Mean, Median, and Mode

> Group #A: There are 200 individuals in a study that describes blood glucose levels. The data show that the blood glucose values seem to be normally distributed (see Introduction) from 50 to 150 mg/mL. That is, there are persons with low values, mid-values, and high values. If the data are plotted, they show a bell-shaped curve that is normally distributed (Figure 1.1).
>
> Group #B: There are also 200 individuals from a different area and the distribution of blood glucose levels is assessed. In this group, it can be noted that about two-thirds of persons have very low glucose values (<50 mg/mL), while the upper third have very high levels (>150 mg/mL); there are very few persons with mid-range glucose values.

Interpretation of the mean and median in the two groups: when Groups A and B are combined, Population 1 appears to have HbA1c levels that are

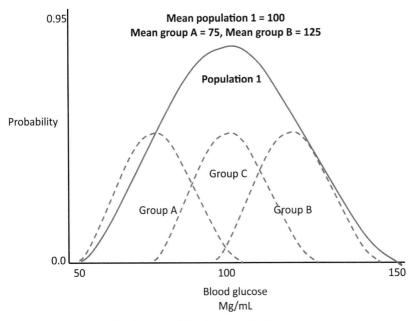

Figure 1.1 Dissimilar distributions of blood glucose levels.

normally distributed; the median is central and likely lies very close to the mean of 100. So, seeing that the population data are normally distributed, one may automatically consider running parametric analyses. However, when broken into Groups A and B and C, the group means of Groups A and B (i.e., 75 and 125), and likely their group medians, have shifted away from the population mean of 100 and the group distributions also appear to be statistically different from each other. Another visual observation is that Group C is likely not statistically different from Groups A and B. In this situation, a non-parametric statistic should be considered when the distributions of blood glucose in Groups A, B, or C are not normally distributed after being stratified from the population, even though the distribution of Population 1 appears to be normally distributed.

In summary, the characteristics of data are extremely important to understand, and therefore simple measures should not be used exclusively; other statistical tools must be considered to fully and correctly describe the data. These include the standard deviation, the coefficient of variation, the range, and the interquartile range.

1.5.4   Range

The lowest number and the highest number of a sorted distribution designates the **range** of the distribution. Ranges are useful when speaking of normal and abnormal ranges for a biological characteristic.

Calculation of the range:

Example for the Clinician

Using the Measured Blood Loss distribution in Table 1.2, the smallest number in the distribution of numbers is 1.50 and the largest number is 68.83. That is the range of values in the Measured Blood Loss distribution.

1.5.5   Interquartile Range

The **interquartile range** (IQR) is at the 25th and 75th percentile of the distribution. This is a useful set of numbers because it presents a little more information about how the data are distributed at a more granular level than the range. In normal situations, the 25th and 75th percentiles of distributions may not be conveniently obvious, as is shown in Figure 1.2,

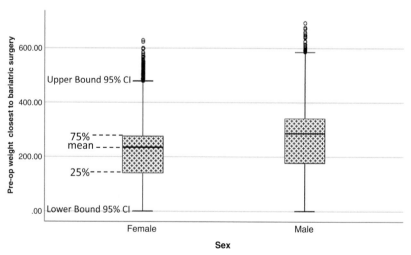

Figure 1.2 Boxplot showing comparison of weight loss by gender.

where we must make decisions on where these distributional demarcations are, as shown in the example below.

Calculation of the IQR:

Example for the Clinician

Again using the distribution of Measured Blood Loss (Table 1.2), the 25th percentile lies somewhere between 1.78 and 3.55 (mean ~ 2.66). The 75th percentile is a judgment call in this case; since the cumulative percentage 73.9% is closer to the 75th percentile than is 78.3%, we can take the MBL value at the 73.9% value and take an MBL value of 8.02 to demarcate the 75th percentile of the distribution. Thus, 2.66–8.02 is the IQR of the distribution.

One of the more informative plots is the **boxplot** (Figure 1.2), which shows the 25th and 75th distributions, the means, the upper and lower bounds of the 95% confidence intervals, and the points outside the 95% confidence interval, which are otherwise known as "outliers." Boxplots are particularly informational and are attractive representations for illustrating statistical differences in journal articles.

Evidently, males were not significantly heavier than females at 24 months post-surgery, as can be determined by the overlap in confidence intervals (Section 3.2).

Knowing these basic statistical calculations and permutations can lead to a broader understanding of your data in terms of their distributions. This understanding is a crucial element in choosing the correct statistical approach. Know your data!

1.5.6   Skewness

Non-normally distributed data do not resemble a bell-shaped curve but rather, they may be skewed to the left or to the right as shown in Figure 1.3. **Skewness** is a term referring to the tail of the distribution, whether it leads off to the right or the left. The skewness of a data distribution refers to the symmetry of the values around the mean of the distribution.

Why do we care about skewness? Because it shows us if the data are normally distributed and therefore, when we should and should not use

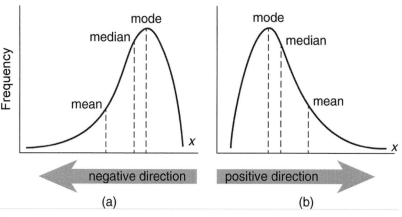

Figure 1.3 Depiction of negative and positive skewness.

parametric analysis techniques. When the mean is equal to the median (is normally distributed), the value for skewness is 0, and is therefore appropriate for parametric analyses. When the majority of values in your distribution are concentrated together at the right or the left, the tail falls off to the right or the left and is therefore called "skewed to the right" or "skewed to the left," respectively, as shown in Figure 1.3, and it is not appropriate for parametric analyses. Skewness values between −2 and 2 are generally acceptable for demonstrating that data are normally distributed, but values less than −2 and greater than 2 are good indications of skewness, or they are not normally distributed, and again, are not good candidates for parametric analyses. For an online skewness calculator, you can enter your data in a tool.[2]

Notice that when data are positively skewed, the mode and the median lie to the left of the mean, while in negatively skewed data, the median and the mode lie to the right of the mean.

The following is a perfect case in point. Presented in Figure 1.4(a) is a frequency distribution and in Figure 1.4(b) a bar chart of a continuous variable: "Days of Hospital Stay." Upon visual scrutiny, this continuous variable is skewed to the left, since most cases stayed 0 or 1 day; thus, Days of Hospital Stay is not normally distributed around the mean. Also, in the cumulative frequency column of the table, you can see that 79.9% of the sample had a length of hospital stay of 2 days or less. Now, had you assumed that Length of Hospital Stay was normally distributed and you ran it through a parametric procedure, your result would be erroneous

(a)

Days of Hospital Stay	Frequency	Percent	Valid percent	Cumulative percent
0	3097	36.9	44.5	44.6
1	1475	17.6	21.2	65.8
2	979	11.7	14.1	79.9
3	390	4.6	5.6	85.5
4	209	2.5	3.0	88.5
5	151	1.8	2.2	90.7
6	123	1.5	1.8	92.4
7	102	1.2	1.5	93.9
8	62	0.7	0.9	94.8
9	60	0.7	0.9	95.6
10	42	0.5	0.6	96.3
11	30	0.4	0.4	96.7
12	24	0.3	0.3	97.0
13	28	0.3	0.4	97.4

(b)

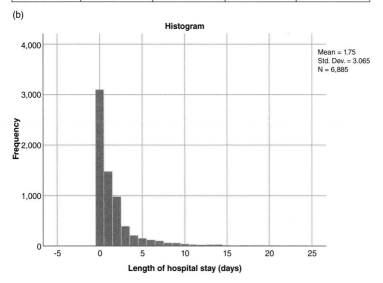

Figure 1.4 (a) Frequency distribution and (b) bar chart of non-normally distributed data.

since it neglects the assumption of distributional normality where skew is equal to zero. More information is available on normality.[3] As an alternative to transforming the data to assume a normal distribution, it is advisable to use non-parametric techniques (Chapter 5).

So, by entering your data into the calculator,[4] the skewness is 2.45, which exceeds the 2 boundary and is thus a candidate for non-parametric analyses, since it would not be possible to transform the data as they do not take on any sort of predictable distribution, such as a logarithmic distribution (Section 2.2).

1.5.7   Kurtosis

Again, examining the distribution of your data before assuming normality is essential when considering whether or not to perform parametric or non-parametric techniques for analysis. Measuring the **kurtosis** of your data is another way to examine the shape of the distribution of your data. As shown in Figure 1.5, kurtosis is specifically a measure of the tails of your distribution. You can see that the tails intercept the x-axis rather sharply (where $\sigma = 1$) or more gently (where $\sigma = 3$). If $\sigma = 3$, your data are normally distributed. If σ is greater than 3 or less than 3, your data are said to be kurtotic, i.e., non-normal. Notice that when you run your data through the

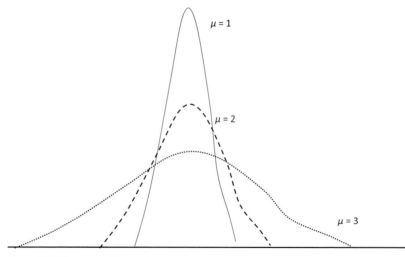

Figure 1.5 Measures of kurtosis.

skewness calculator,[5] it also generates a value for kurtosis. You may use these values to decide if your data are or are not normally distributed and apply the appropriate set of statistics accordingly, i.e., parametric or non-parametric.

1.6   Frequency Distributions

In Table 1.2 we examined the distribution of Measured Blood Loss during surgery. This is called a **frequency distribution** of all data points in my data file. When a statistician receives a new dataset, the first exploratory analysis they often run is a frequency distribution as a first step to check the data for accuracy and coding errors. They may run "frequencies" on all variables in the dataset. The utility of the frequency distribution is that one can easily identify values that are out of range and values that are character instead of numeric, or vice versa. One may also run frequency distributions to find meaningful cutoffs if one wishes to categorize these variables by the mean, the median, or the 25th percentiles – e.g., age (0–2, 3–5, 6–12), weight (90–100, 100–150, 150–200), etc. These are common data transformations that are made to continuous values before entering the newly coded variables into other analyses.

For example, see Table 1.3.

Table 1.3   Utility of frequency distributions

	Race	Frequency	Percent	Valid percent	Cumulative percent
Valid	0.0	5	0.1	0.1	0.1
	1.0 Caucasian	4656	67.7	68.0	68.0
	2.0 African American	1854	27.0	27.1	95.1
	3.0 Asian	71	1.0	1.0	96.1
	4.0 Hispanic	161	2.3	2.4	98.5
	5.0 Other	101	1.5	1.5	100.0
	6.0	2	0.0	0.0	100.0
	9.0	1	0.0	0.0	100.0
	Total	6851	99.6	100.0	
Missing	System	25	0.4		
Total		**6876**	**100.0**		

By running a frequency distribution, you can note in Table 1.3 that the 0s, 6s, and 9s are errors and that race is missing for 25 records in your raw data. This simple table should prompt the data crew to find these missing values and complete them, and also find the records containing the errors and fix them. This process is known as "cleaning your data."

Frequency Distribution

Moving from left to right in Table 1.4, the value in the first column is the actual value for number of post-surgical complications.

Table 1.4 How to interpret a frequency distribution table

Number of post-surgical complications	Frequency	Percent	Valid percent	Cumulative percent
0	6420	76.4	97.7	97.7
1	131	1.6	2.0	99.7
2	16	0.2	0.2	100.0
3	1	0.0	0.0	100.0
Total	6568	78.2	100.0	
Missing	1832	21.8		
Total	**8400**	**100.0**		

The **frequency** represents the number of times the value appears in the dataset. The **percent** column shows the proportion of that value within the whole distribution, including those with missing values. There are 8400 total records in the database, of which 1832 are missing values for number of post-surgical complications. The **valid percent** shows the proportion of that value in your database when you *exclude* missing values. And finally, the **cumulative percent** shows the increasing (or cumulative) percentage of values from the lowest value in the distribution to the highest value (0% to 100%). When reporting frequencies in manuscripts or reports, it is best to state the total number of records in the database, the number of missing values, and the valid percentage of values in the dataset.

Because Estimated Blood Loss (EBL) is a continuous value (Table 1.5), one would tend to examine the mean and standard deviation of EBL,

Table 1.5 A frequency distribution of Estimated Blood Loss

Estimated Blood Loss (in dL)	Frequency	Percent	Valid percent	Cumulative percent
100.00	1	4.3	4.3	4.3
150.00	3	13.0	13.0	17.4
200.00	1	4.3	4.3	21.7
300.00	4	17.4	17.4	39.1
400.00	3	13.0	13.0	52.2
450.00	1	4.3	4.3	56.5
500.00	4	17.4	17.4	73.9
800.00	2	8.7	8.7	82.6
1000.00	2	8.7	8.7	91.3
1100.00	1	4.3	4.3	95.7
6250.00	1	4.3	4.3	100.0
Total	**23**	**100.0**	**100.0**	

Table 1.6 Making clinically relevant stratifications of continuous data

EBL (dL)	Mean baseline weight	SD	P
≤200	214.53	10.22	
201–400	220.64	12.32	<0.001
401–500	228.43	10.56	
≥501	258.22	13.65	

which is an appropriate way to summarize normally distributed, continuous data.

For example, look at mean weight compared across categories of EBL groupings of the EBL distribution (Table 1.6). When grouped into such clinically meaningful quartiles, i.e., ≤200, 201–400, 401–500, 501+, you can then use these categories to compare another continuous variable, say, the mean baseline weight between these EBL categories to answer the question: Do patients who lose more blood during surgery weigh more than those who lose less blood?

So, the importance of this example is to show the utility of frequency distributions and how they can aid in the manipulative grouping of data in order to conduct meaningful statistical analyses.

1.7   Measures of Dispersion and Variance

1.7.1   Standard Deviation

The standard deviation is one way to describe the variation of your data in relation to the mean of your data. It is a sum of the difference between each data point and the sample mean divided by the number of records in your dataset. The distance of each value from the mean is squared to ensure we do not obtain negative values, since the standard deviation must always be an integer whether it be lower or higher than the mean. Later, we take the square root of this difference divided by n, to negate the squaring:

$$\sigma = \sqrt{\frac{\sum (x - \bar{x})^2}{n}}$$

where

σ = standard deviation
$\sum$ = sum of
x = each value in the dataset
$\bar{x}$ = mean of all values in the dataset
n = number of values in the dataset.

Calculation of the standard deviation:

What is the standard deviation of 2, 3, 6, and 10?
Answer: Firstly, find the mean of these four values:

$2 + 3 + 6 + 10 = 21$
$21/4 = 5.25$

$$SD = \sqrt{\frac{(2 - 5.25)^2 + (3 - 5.25)^2 + (6 - 5.25)^2 + (10 - 5.25)^2}{4}}$$

$$= \sqrt{\frac{10.56 + 5.06 + 0.56 + 22.56}{4}}$$

$$= \sqrt{9.685} = 3.11.$$

It might be more intuitive to make the calculations of the standard deviation in tabular form, as shown in the next example.

Standard Deviation

Table 1.7 shows the temperature in a very hot African city over a 20-day period and the 20-day average (mean) temperature for the 20 consecutive days.

Table 1.7 Calculation of standard deviation

	Close	20-Day mean	Deviation	Deviation squared
1	109.00	112.30	−3.30	10.91
2	103.06	112.30	−9.24	85.38
3	102.75	112.30	−9.55	91.26
4	108.00	112.30	−4.30	18.52
5	107.56	112.30	−4.74	22.47
6	105.25	112.30	−7.05	49.75
7	107.69	112.30	−4.62	21.30
8	108.63	112.30	−3.68	13.53
9	107.00	112.30	−5.30	28.12
10	109.00	112.30	−3.30	10.91
11	110.00	112.30	−2.30	5.30
12	112.75	112.30	0.45	0.20
13	113.50	112.30	1.20	1.43
14	114.25	112.30	1.95	3.79
15	115.25	112.30	2.95	8.68
16	121.50	112.30	9.20	84.58
17	126.88	112.30	14.57	212.34
18	122.50	112.30	10.20	103.97
19	119.00	112.30	6.70	44.85
20	122.50	112.30	10.20	103.97
	2246.06	112.30		921.28
				DevSqr/20 46.06
				StdDev 6.787

To calculate the standard deviation, the distance of each daily temperature from the mean temperature is calculated and then "squared" to obtain a positive value for the negative deviations from the mean. These squared distances are then summed together and divided by the n of your sample. Then, the square root of that value is taken to normalize the squared value back to the unsquared value (the correction).

1.7.2   Standard Error

The standard error is a value that pertains to the variance of the population mean, not the sample mean! Mathematically, it is $SD/\sqrt{n}$. Conceptually, it is a measure of how precise a parameter is in the population. That parameter can be the mean or the correlation coefficient (Section 4.3.3). If we were to repeatedly pull samples from the same population and measure the mean weight for each sample, the SE of all the repeated weight measurements is the measure of precision of all sample mean estimates.

1.7.3   Coefficient of Variation

The coefficient of variation (CV) is another measure that describes the dispersion of measurements in terms of the standard deviation from the mean. It is commonly used in reproducibility and repeatability studies to determine how steady the measurements are (or are not) from an identical sample or person. Usually, if you are repeatedly testing the same sample over and over, it is preferred that the value for the CV is small. The CV is calculated by dividing the standard deviation by the mean of a distribution which is derived from the same sample or subject. It is just an expression used to show the ratio of the standard deviation from the mean.

CV for a sample:

$$CV = \frac{SD}{\bar{x}} \times 100\%$$

where SD is the standard deviation and $\bar{x}$ is the sample mean.

Using the values above, the mean (5.25) and standard deviation (3.11) give a CV of 0.59, or 59%, which is quite high. Keep in mind that this calculation of CV is only appropriate for normally distributed measurement data, meaning that one would not normally calculate a mean or standard deviation or CV for heavily skewed data (Section 1.5.6).

Calculation of the coefficient of variation:

Example for the Laboratorian

Laboratory A and Laboratory B have each been given 10 replicate aliquots of blood from *one healthy volunteer* to test for blood glucose. Both labs performed their tests using the same measurement procedure, used the same tester, the same measuring instrument under the same conditions, in the same location, and the test repetition occurred over a short period of time.

Laboratory A gets a mean of 81.1 and SD of 15.7.
Laboratory B gets a mean of 82.5 and SD of 20.4.

Which lab had better test repeatability?

Laboratory A CV $= 15.7/81.1 \times 100 = 19.35\%$.
Laboratory B CV $= 20.4/82.5 \times 100 = 24.73\%$.

Clearly, Laboratory A had less variation in blood glucose levels in relation to the mean value, and thus had better test repeatability.

CVs are also computed when reproducibility or precision (Section 8.3.3) of one test is being assessed for variation. Ideally, the CV of a test should not change if tested in two different labs; that is, the one test should perform identically in both labs.

Links to Online Tools

[1] www.mayo.edu/research/documents/parametric-and-nonparametric-demystifying-the-terms/doc-20408960

[2] www.socscistatistics.com/tests/skewness/default.aspx

[3] www.wessa.net/rwasp_skewness_kurtosis.wasp#output

[4] www.socscistatistics.com/tests/skewness/default.aspx

[5] www.socscistatistics.com/tests/skewness/default.aspx

2 Types of Data and their Distributions

It is imperative that you know what type of data you are analyzing to know what type of statistical procedure to use. In this section, we will be examining two classes of data: continuous and non-continuous.

2.1 Continuous Data

Weight and height are examples of **continuous data**. They have a quantitative range from a low value to a high value, a mean, median, and mode, quartiles, and 95% confidence intervals.

2.1.1 Normally Distributed Continuous Data

Normally distributed continuous data (or variables) are normally distributed, meaning that their values tend to follow a "bell-shaped" distribution such as that seen below. One should never assume that their data are normally distributed, which is why one must always run frequency distributions and plots of their data. The reason one should avoid making an automatic assumption of normality is because we want to avoid applying the incorrect statistical technique (such as a T-test or a Pearson correlation) that assumes the data follow a normal distribution; such techniques are referred to as "parametric" analyses (Section 1.4). More information is available on parametric analyses.[6]

You can note in the histogram in Figure 2.1 that the age in this sample is normally distributed, i.e., bell-shaped, and thus is an eligible variable for a parametric statistical procedure.

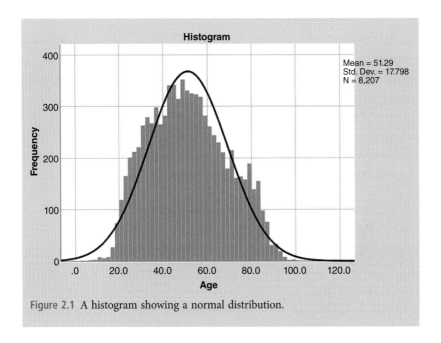

Figure 2.1 A histogram showing a normal distribution.

2.1.2   Non-normally Distributed Continuous Data

As described in Sections 1.5.6 (skewness) and 1.5.7 (kurtosis), the distribution of your data can be assessed by visually inspecting the distribution, or by calculating the skewness and kurtosis of your data. Data may be transformed into a normal distribution in any number of ways, depending on how the data are distributed. One may see data that are heavily skewed to the left or to the right, in which case non-parametric analyses should be considered. However, if the data visually appear to follow some predictable pattern, one may transform them to see if conformation to a normal distribution is possible.

2.2   Log-distributed Data

Data distributions that increase in unequal intervals, e.g., from 1 to 10 to 100 to 1000 and onward (**log$_{10}$ distribution**), are called log$_{10}$-distributed data. These are not normally distributed; thus, one would not be interested in the mean or the variance of the data because it wouldn't tell us anything useful about its distribution. For the same reason, one would not perform a parametric analysis on log-distributed data. Of course, there are different rates of increase in biological processes. One may show a doubling of values, i.e., 1 ➜ 2 ➜ 4 ➜ 8 ➜, etc. (which looks like a **natural log**), while another may show a tripling of quantities, i.e., 1 ➜ 3 ➜ 9 ➜ 27, etc. Again, if it is your aim to conduct a parametric analysis of your data, you will need to first decide what kind of distribution you have in your data and then "normalize" it by taking the natural log or the $\log_{10}$ of your values and use that "transformed" value in your parametric analysis.

2.2.1 $\log_{10}$-distributed Data

HIV viral load data, for example, are $\log_{10}$-distributed data, as are distributions of other viral species such as Hepatitis B and C, among others. Detectable HIV RNA copies/mL range from 50 copies/mL (lower limit of detection on most assays) to approximately 10 million copies/mL; these data are not normally distributed. If you attempt to plot these values, you will quickly find it difficult to extend the y-axis far enough to accommodate

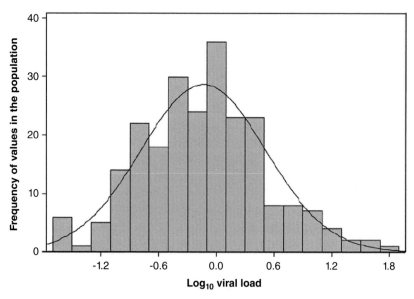

Figure 2.2 Histogram showing $\log_{10}$-transformed data. Source.[7]

values ranging from 10 through 10,000,000. Thus, before applying parametric techniques to such variables, one must $\log_{10}$ transform the distribution to make the values approximate a normal distribution. So, when you transform a $\log_{10}$ distribution such as this, 50 to 10 million, you will see that the transformed values of the $\log_{10}$ distribution are almost normally distributed, as shown in Figure 2.2.

$\log_{10}$-distributed Data

When looking at a frequency distribution of HIV viral load data, it is easy to see that it is $\log_{10}$ distributed. To transform HIV viral load for parametric analyses, one must take $\log_{10}$ of the viral load and use that value for parametric analysis (Table 2.1).

Table 2.1 $\log_{10}$-distributed data

HIV viral load (copies/mL) (non-normally distributed)	$\log_{10}$ HIV viral load (normalized data)
7	0.845
210	2.32
3,400	3.53
15,601	4.19
550,671	5.74
3,089,900	6.49
40,898,383	7.61

You may find $\log_{10}$ of any number using an online $\log_{10}$ calculator.[8]

2.2.2   Natural Log-distributed Data

This is something that mathematicians have a difficult time explaining to the curious student. However, getting stuck at this point will surely limit understanding of future statistical concepts that rely on its understanding.

In nature, life takes time and growth to reach its limit and capacity on Earth. Each species of bacteria, plants, and animals have varying rates of growth and reproduction. Figure 2.3 shows this relationship between progression and the time it takes to reach endpoints. The reason this is

	Logarithms = Time	Exponents = Growth
Time/Growth Perspective	$\ln(x)$ *Time needed to grow to x* *(with 100% continuous compounding)*	e^x *Amount of growth after time x* *(with 100% continuous compounding)*

Figure 2.3 Time/growth perspective.

important to point out in a statistics book now is because if one recognizes the geometric nature of increase, one will know how to transform the data to a normally distributed variable.

e^x = Amount of growth of bacterial cells, e.g., after a fixed time period (x). So, for example, the amount of growth for two bacterial cells to reach 32 cells is 2^4 ($2 \rightarrow 4 \rightarrow 8 \rightarrow 16 \rightarrow 32$).

$\log x$ ($\ln(x)$) = Amount of time to reach sufficient number of bacterial cells for my experiment. $\ln(x)$ is the time needed to grow from two cells to 32 cells.

Bacterial Growth

In the laboratory, under favorable conditions, a growing bacterial sample doubles at regular intervals. Growth is by geometric progression: 1, 2, 4, 8, etc. or $2^0, 2^1, 2^2, 2^3, \ldots, 2^n$ (where n = number of generations). This is called **exponential growth**. So, in this case, the exponent is 2^n.

Again, why do we want to normalize our logarithmically distributed data if we can? *Answer:* parametric analyses are, for the most part, more robust than non-parametric analyses. Parametric analyses use the actual data values whereas non-parametric analyses use ranks as proxies to the actual values in the data distribution.

2.2.3   Geometric Mean Titer

A researcher is conducting a combination vaccine trial in control subjects who are on the standard vaccine, and the exploratory subjects are on the standard vaccine plus an experimental vaccine.

Before calculating sample size for this trial, one must clearly express the alternative and null hypotheses.

Table 2.2   How to calculate the geometric mean titer

Number of sera	Antibody titer
1	8
1	32
1	64
1	128
1	2,563
1	51,256
1	204,823
Total = 7	Product = 5.642×10^{19}
	$\sqrt[7]{5.642 \times 10^{19}} = 663.19 = $ GMT

Alternative hypothesis. The exploratory combination vaccine (exploratory plus standard vaccine) produces an antibody response that is three times greater than the standard vaccine.

Null hypothesis. The combination vaccine produces an antibody response that is non-inferior, or no better or worse than the standard vaccine.

Of course, antibody response is expressed on a log scale. How will we calculate the mean antibody titer for each group to compare these groups when the data are log distributed?

As discussed earlier, one would need to transform or normalize the values to approximate a normal distribution. How is this achieved? Walking through Table 2.2, this is achieved by:

- Multiplying all of the antibody titers together: $8 \times 32 \times 64 \times \cdots \times$ 204,823 = product.
- Taking the *n*th root of that product: $\sqrt[n]{\text{product}}$ (*n* = # specimens). We have seven antibody titer measures, so geometric mean titer (GMT) = $\sqrt[7]{\text{product}}$.

So, why would we want to know the mean of these two logarithmic distributions? We do this to describe the central tendency of this logarithmic distribution, or more simply, the mean and standard deviation of the distribution so we can make reasonable comparisons of antibody responses to the vaccine arms.

Understandably, you wouldn't want to have to do this manually for a large number of titers, so you can plug your numbers into an online calculator.[9]

Geometric Mean Titer

Let's say, for example, that you are making serial dilutions of serum to quantify the amount (titer) of HIV in a patient. To do this, it is important to make careful titrations so that the end-product is representative of its source, i.e., the patient's blood.

2.3   Non-continuous Data

Non-continuous variables have discrete values that code for a characteristic. The characteristics can be semi-quantitative (binary and ordinal) or completely without quantitative value (nominal). Generally, they do not carry units of measurement. The word "dichotomous" is interchangeable with "binary", i.e., there are only two choices – such as positive or negative.

2.3.1   Binary or Dichotomous Data

Binary data have two values. The values of binary data can take on two forms; they can be quasi-ordinal, such as 0 and 1 for absence and presence of disease, respectively, or binary variables can take on nominal values such as 1 and 2 for male and female, respectively. These data types have no units of measurement and the values assigned to these binary variables should be well documented so that you know how to interpret your results.

2.3.2   Ordinal Data

Think of "order." **Ordinal variables** take on a semi-quantitative value; as the value increases, the result is better or worse. Another example is the Likert scale, which usually ranges from 1 to 5, where 1 = strongly disagree, 2 = disagree, 3 = neutral, 4 = agree, and 5 = strongly agree. Although semi-quantitative, ordinal variables are not measured in any tangible units.

2.3.3   Nominal Data

Nominal variables have no logical, quantitative value, so codes must be clearly documented (see Table 2.3). An example might be gender: 1 = male,

Table 2.3 An example of a frequency distribution of a nominal variable: "Patient Status"

	n	Percent	Cumulative percent
1 = Inpatient	37,488	92.42	92.4
2 = Office Visit	1,728	4.26	96.7
3 = Outpatient	1,242	3.06	99.7
4 = SD Clinic	102	0.26	100.0
Total	**40,560**	**100.0**	

2 = female, which by nature appears to be a binary variable. Again, nominal data are not measured in quantifiable units.

So, why is it important to know about your data? Knowing the distribution of your data is paramount as the distribution predicts, or rather dictates, the correct analytic technique which must be employed to analyze your data. Without knowing if your data are normally distributed, it would be too easy to perform the incorrect analysis and, thereby, produce erroneous results.

Links to Online Tools

[6] www.statsref.com/HTML/index.html?normal_distribution.html
[7] http://teachersinstitute.yale.edu/curriculum/units/2009/4/09.04.07.x.html
[8] www.miniwebtool.com/log-base-10-calculator/
[9] www.alcula.com/calculators/statistics/geometric-mean/

3   Significance Testing

3.1   Multiple Comparisons

Scientists are a curious breed. They seek knowledge to advance science to improve health and innovate novel therapies and techniques. Most scientists will develop hypotheses and gather evidence to support or refute their scientific suspicions or hypotheses. Therefore, analysis of the data should be intentional and directed at the research question in hand.

However, sometimes, scientists may "explore" the data for a multitude of associations, correlations, and significant findings. This practice, otherwise known as a "fishing expedition," is generally frowned upon among the scientific community, because some statistically significant findings may be significant by chance alone, i.e., the findings are random.

In Section 3.2, we will touch on the topic of accepting statistical significance at the $P \leq 0.05$ level. This means that we accept that two samples are statistically and significantly different with respect to age, for example, even though up to 5% of their age distributions overlap. Further, this means that 1 in 20 (5%) values can be in the same area of the age distribution by chance; that is allowed and is still considered significantly different.

However, what that also means is that if you run multiple "exploratory" analyses, 1 in 20 comparisons may well show statistically significant results by chance alone. Would you report these significant results?

What is the obligation of the scientist in reporting on these phenomena? The scientist must first avoid these fishing expeditions, but for those who truly have many, many data points to analyze to address a hypothesis, one simple tactic to apply is called a **Bonferroni correction**. This is simply the lowering of the threshold for significance by setting P-values (see Section 3.2) for significance from 0.05 to 0.01 or 0.001, if we are getting into 20 or more comparisons, as shown in Table 3.1.

Table 3.1   Example of making multiple comparisons

	Patients with:	N	Mean	Std. dev.	P-value
Age	No stones	764	52.306	17.9147	0.616
	Stones	4281	52.670	18.5940	
Length of hospital	No stones	753	79.52	194.477	0.456
stay (hours)	Stones	4199	55.75	121.375	
Length of hospital	No stones	753	54.92	151.371	<0.001
stay post-op	Stones	4199	37.71	103.160	
Incision start time	No stones	222	12:21:28.92	3:42:53.066	<0.001
	Stones	1364	12:40:54.99	3:52:10.779	
Incision close time	No stones	221	16:38:56.20	41:24:36.58	0.245
	Stones	1357	14:08:22.42	4:56:33.200	
Duration of	No stones	127	1:45:51.97	4:27:25.130	0.032
operation	Stones	819	43:27:34.43	12:02:03.53	
Time of conversion	No stones	3	15:13:40.00	7:09:28.609	0.696
	Stones	12	14:49:05.00	5:24:50.162	
	Stones	1449	78.50	14.614	
Estimated blood	No stones	690	79.897	201.8501	0.002
loss (mL)	Stones	3978	61.841	131.0781	
Gallstone size,	No stones	18	8.9333	7.99470	0.002
ultrasound	Stones	339	15.1074	8.26658	
(quantitative)					
Gallbladder wall	No stones	139	5.2071	2.96172	0.015
width,	Stones	1030	4.6148	2.64147	
ultrasound					
(quantitative)					
Diameter of	No stones	358	4.7199162010	2.45170203100	0.018
common bile	Stones	2287	5.0598513330	2.52597047400	
duct, ultrasound					
(mm)					
Wall thickness by	No stones	3	4.667	3.5119	0.862
CT (mm)	Stones	34	4.300	3.4754	
	Stones	205	7.4355	3.62446	
EFHIDA – ejection	No stones	255	17.4071	18.50824	<0.001
fraction (%)	Stones	401	27.1761	27.02899	
TTGB – time to	No stones	302	64.146	286.9939	0.311
gallbladder	Stones	767	91.785	438.1906	
visualization	Stones	643	72.236	223.1638	
(min)	Stones	4725	0.04	0.201	

Table 3.1 (cont.)

	Patients with:	N	Mean	Std. dev.	P-value
PostopERCP – post-operative ERCP	No stones	838	0.01	0.119	0.193
	Stones	4721	0.02	0.144	
Polypcm – maximal diameter of polyp (cm)	No stones	19	0.5053	1.11827	0.003
	Stones	88	0.0801	0.32159	
Polyp	No stones	52	0.246	0.5143	0.002
	Stones	224	0.076	0.2973	
	Stones	4782	0.19	0.389	
White blood cells (1000s/uL)	No stones	557	9.35473	4.375053	0.634
	Stones	3204	9.46214	5.003479	
Blood urea nitrogen (mg/dL)	No stones	548	15.2281	12.01526	0.032
	Stones	3130	14.1313	10.85563	
	Stones	47	38.2606	113.04491	
Aspartate transferase (U/L)	No stones	443	63.219	151.5821	0.215
	Stones	2556	72.095	136.7873	
Alanine transferase (U/L)	No stones	443	66.271	144.1343	0.040
	Stones	2556	81.499	143.7652	
Alkaline phosphatase (U/L)	No stones	460	105.974	87.7522	0.324
	Stones	2565	110.431	89.4549	
	Stones	2055	0.3599221	1.01814111	
Albumin (g/dL)	No stones	434	3.7308	0.78650	0.266
	Stones	2521	3.7886	1.03143	
Prothrombin time (s)	No stones	343	12.4836734700	6.65885256400	0.012
	Stones	1979	11.8154421400	4.03779250400	
Internat'l normalized ratio	No stones	341	1.43328	5.244791	0.034
	Stones	1967	1.13654	1.370047	
Heart rate at triage in ER or in office pre-op visit	No stones	175	82.3960	16.00489	0.009
	Stones	1063	78.8646	16.50805	

If we set the *P*-value (Section 3.2) at ≤ 0.05, two or three of these 26 *T*-tests for differences may have been accepted as being significantly different, when in the real world they have no biological relationship whatsoever! By lowering the criteria for significance to 0.01, we lose six associations (dark gray) but at the 0.01 level, we retain nine associations (light gray), which are more likely to be real biologic associations.

3.2   Confidence Intervals vs. *P*-values

Oftentimes, scientists may regard the *P*-value as the definitive validation of significance, while statisticians usually prefer seeing the confidence intervals because they provide a visual tool that identifies the divergence or overlap of distributions from two or more groups, or how far apart (or significantly different) they are.

3.2.1 Confidence Intervals

A **confidence interval** around a proportion or a mean shows the distribution of values in your sample into which the majority (usually set at 95%) of values in the population will fall (the population from which the sample is drawn). You can set any level of confidence, depending on the stringency of your proposed goal, e.g., at 80%, 90%, 95%, or 99%. If you set the level at 95%, the 95% confidence interval is the boundaries within which 95% of your values will reside in the universe or population.

The calculation of confidence intervals can be done in several ways. Here we focus on those calculated for continuous variables (weight, height, blood glucose levels, etc.) and for proportions (likely prevalence of disease, sensitivity, specificity, etc.).

For example, what does a *P*-value of 0.034 tell us about the distribution and variability of weight between two groups, such as those with and without diabetes? It tells us that the probability that this association is due to chance is less than 5%, but it doesn't say anything about the distributions of weight in the two groups. However, what does the following information provide?

Group A Diabetics: Mean weight 230 lbs (95% CI = 180.45 − 250.62).
Group B Non-diabetics: Mean weight 150 lbs (95% CI = 143.23 − 172.11).

Well, it tells us that:

- If you were to make 100 measurements of weight in diabetics you would expect 95% of these measurements to fall within the window of 180.45–250.62, and for 100 measurements in non-diabetics, 95% of weight values will fall within the range of 143.23–172.11.

- In each distribution, 5% (2.5% lower bound, 2.5% upper bound) of the values will fall outside of these lower and upper bounds, because these 95% confidence intervals are an estimate of the true 95% confidence interval in the universe, and you have merely drawn samples from the universe of diabetics and non-diabetics.
- This also tells us that these confidence intervals do not overlap whatsoever, and the difference between them is statistically significant.
- If the 95% confidence intervals do overlap, such as A: 180.45–250.62 vs. B: 155.05–181.22, they are not statistically different.

There is one more piece of information you will need to calculate the confidence intervals, and that is the Z-score. Z is a constant taken from a table of Z-scores; it represents the number of standard deviation units from the mean that serve as the lower and upper bounds of the confidence intervals. You will see the symbols $Z_{1/\alpha}$, which is simply the Z-score that corresponds to where you are setting α. We select different Z-scores depending on how precise we want the calculation to be, but in general and depending on the desired width of your confidence interval, researchers commonly use three to four Z-scores, as shown below:

CI	α	Z-score
90%	0.10	1.64
95%	0.05	1.96
98%	0.02	2.33
99%	0.01	2.58

Calculating Confidence Intervals for Proportions

$$p \pm Z_{1-\alpha/2}\sqrt{\frac{p(1-p)}{n}}$$

where

p = the proportion, like sensitivity = 0.98 (not to be confused with the P-value)

$Z_{1-\alpha/2}$ = the Z-value corresponding to a 95% CI = 1.96 [$Z_{1-\alpha/2}$ is simply the Z-score associated with (1−0.05/2), which represents the 95% CI]

n = the number of test results in the sample.

So, if the sensitivity or specificity of a test is 98% (or 0.98) and $n = 200$:

$$95\% \text{ CI} = 0.98 \pm 1.96\sqrt{\frac{0.98(1 - 0.98)}{200}}$$
$$= 0.98 \pm 1.96\sqrt{0.000098}$$
$$= 0.98 \pm 1.96 \times 0.0099$$
$$= 0.98 \pm 0.0194$$
$$= 0.9606 - 0.9994.$$

Distance between lower and upper bounds = 0.0388.

Now, let's tighten the confidence interval to 99%, where the Z-score is 2.58, and calculate the confidence intervals again:

$$99\% \text{ CI} = 0.98 \pm 2.58\sqrt{\frac{0.98(1 - 0.98)}{200}}$$
$$= 0.98 \pm 2.58\sqrt{0.000098}$$
$$= 0.98 \pm 2.58 \times 0.0099$$
$$= 0.98 \pm 0.0255$$
$$= 0.9545 - 1.0000.$$

Distance between lower and upper bounds = 0.0455.

So, you can now see that tightening the confidence interval from 95% to 99% changed the interval from a width of 0.0388 to a width of 0.0455, a difference of 0.0067.

Calculating Confidence Intervals for Continuous Variables

To calculate the 95% confidence interval for continuous variables such as weight or height, you need just four pieces of information:

- The mean weight or height (230).
- The N, or sample size (500).
- The standard deviation of weight or height (measuring the variance around the mean) (20.45).
- The Z-score or the selection of the associated confidence interval.

Using the formula:

$95\% \text{ CI} = \bar{x} \pm Z_{1/\alpha} \times \text{standard error } \left(\text{SE} = \text{SD}/\sqrt{N}\right)$

(review Section 1.7.2).

Therefore:

$95\% \text{ CI weight} = \text{mean weight} \pm 1.96(\text{SE}).$

So, using the example above, for this sample:

$$95\% \text{ CI} = 230 \pm 1.96\left(20.45/\sqrt{500}\right)$$
$$= 230 \pm 1.96 \times 20.45/22.36$$
$$= 230 \pm 1.96 \times .91$$
$$= 229.09 - 230.91$$

(these values are called the lower and upper bounds of the 95% confidence interval).

Note that the multiplication factor will be different if one decides to place a 98% or 99% confidence interval, in which case the multiplier will be 2.33 or 2.58, respectively.

Now, if N is very low, the confidence interval will be very wide, since N is in the denominator of the equation for both proportions and continuous data. So, when one sees a graph with very wide and overlapping confidence intervals between groups, as shown in Figure 3.1, this means that there is a large amount of variation in weight loss, giving rise to a large standard error (or, that the sample sizes for the 36-month points are low, relative to earlier points). Now, isn't this more informative than a P-value? One can confidently state that Laparoscopic Roux-en-Y Gastric Bypass (LRYGB)

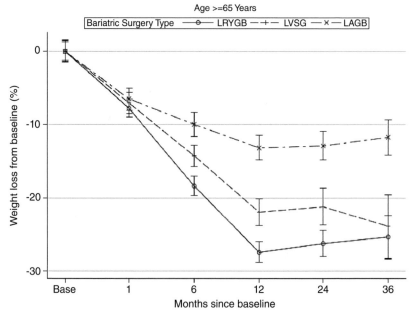

Figure 3.1 The relationship of sample size and the width of the confidence interval.

produced significantly more weight loss at 6, 12, and 24 months (no P-value needed) than Laparoscopic Sleeve Gastrectomy (LVSG) and Laparoscopic Gastric Band (LAGB) procedures, as illustrated in Figure 3.1. One can also confidently say that those who underwent LAGB surgery lost significantly less weight than those who underwent LRYGB and LVSG, because the distributions of their weight loss values are significantly different, i.e., their 95% confidence intervals at 6 through 36 months do not overlap at all.

3.2.2 P-values

P-values represent the probability that comparisons between groups or variables are or are not statistically different or correlated by chance alone. We usually accept significance at $P < 0.05$, or at more stringent levels, e.g., $P < 0.01$. For example, for the statement "patients in Group A were significantly heavier than patients in Group B," $P = 0.043$ means that the chance that this statistically significant finding could have happened by chance alone is <0.05, or $<5\%$.

We allow this 5% **margin of error**, which indicates that if one conducts 20 or more analyses, 1/20 (or 5%) may be statistically significant just by chance alone. Again, when making such multiple comparisons, i.e., ≥ 20 comparisons of, say, differences in clinical features between those with vs. without gall-bladder cancer, 5% of these comparisons would be significantly different by chance alone and may have no clinical relevance. In such cases, one would lower the acceptable P-value to <0.01, so as to avoid stating significance by chance. This maneuver is the Bonferroni correction. Of course, laboratorians and clinicians must honor their clinical expertise to decide if a statistically significant finding is clinically relevant or spurious (see more in Section 3.1).

3.3   Hypotheses (Alternative and Null)

A **hypothesis** is a statement that defends the expected outcome of an investigation. It is an informed presumption that serves as a starting point of a study. You might see the **alternative hypothesis** denoted as H_1 and the **null hypothesis** denoted as H_0. The hypothesis is a statement and is never a question; in fact, by the time you complete testing your hypothesis, you will make an informed decision to accept or reject it based on your findings.

An alternative hypothesis and a null hypothesis must be established. For example, there must be a hypothesis about the performance of a test, let's say before embarking on the calculation of the necessary sample size to determine the true sensitivity of the test. The alternative hypothesis is that Test A is statistically and significantly higher than Test B. The null hypothesis is usually that Test A is no better or is worse than Test B. It completely depends on what effect you are examining. The point is that the alternative and null hypotheses are opposites of each other.

Sample Hypotheses

Alternative hypothesis (H_1): Treatment A is neither better nor worse than the current standard of care treatment.

Null hypothesis (H_0): Treatment A is either worse or better than the current standard of care.

Alternative hypothesis (H_1): The sensitivity of Test A is significantly higher than the sensitivity of Test B.

Null hypothesis (H_0): The sensitivity of Test A is equal to or worse than the sensitivity of Test B.

Alternative hypothesis (H_1): Height and weight are highly correlated (say ≥ 0.5).

Null hypothesis (H_0): Height and weight are not highly correlated (say <0.5).

Alternative hypothesis (H_1): Patients with poorly controlled diabetes have significantly higher HbA1c levels than those with well-controlled diabetes.

Null hypothesis (H_0): The HbA1c levels of patients with poorly controlled diabetes are equal to or worse than for patients with well-controlled diabetes.

3.4   One-Sided vs. Two-Sided Tests

While you develop your hypothesis, you must decide if it is a one-sided hypothesis or a two-sided hypothesis. Choosing a one- or two-tailed test is a choice that depends largely on the nature of the association. It's pretty simple to determine. Think of what you know and don't know about what result you will obtain at the end of your experiment. If you have the preconceived knowledge that error rates in Test A are indeed higher than they are in Test B, you should use a **one-sided test**, meaning that the effect (the error rate) is expected to only go in one direction, i.e., error rates will always be higher in Test A. Naturally, one would likely select to conduct a one-sided test of significance to study the association between height and weight, since they usually increase together in one direction as shown in Figure 3.2. A more obvious example of applying a one-sided test is when you are examining cell viability after being frozen in a $-80°C$ freezer for 3 months. It certainly is not possible for cells to be more than 100% viable, so the one-sided P-value should be reported since the cells are certain to decline in viability, in one direction only.

However, if you don't know whether Test A will have higher or lower error rates than Test B, you may use the more conservative **two-sided test**, meaning that the error rate of Test A can be higher or lower than that of Test B, i.e., the effect might go in either direction.

In this case, we presume that the proportion of false results in Test A is always larger, as determined by past analysis or suspicion. So, we would

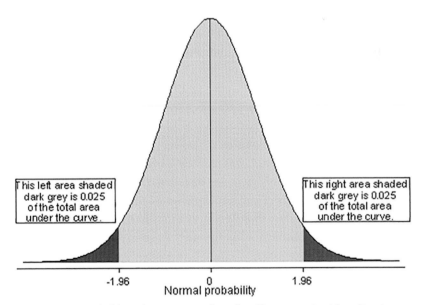

Figure 3.2 Two-sided hypothesis testing where the effect can go in either direction.

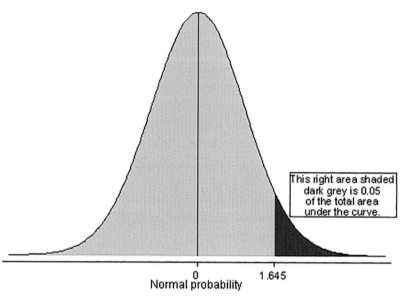

Figure 3.3 One-sided hypothesis testing.

choose the one-sided or one-tailed test. See Figure 3.3 for a visualization of a one-tailed test.

Another example would be if you wanted to test whether age in your sample is significantly different from a fixed number, say 23 years; you would select a two-tailed test since you don't know if age in your sample is greater or less than 23 years – you select both sides of the curve.

The *P*-values associated with one- and two-sided hypothesis tests do differ quantitatively, so be sure to select the correct test and report the correct *P*-value.

If you have preconceived knowledge that error rates in Test A are indeed higher than they are in Test B, you may use a one-sided test, meaning that the effect is expected to only go in one direction, i.e., error rates will always be higher in Test A. However, if you don't know whether Test A will have higher or lower error rates than Test B, you may use the more robust two-sided test, meaning that you allow the effect to go in either direction.

Borrowed from Syque.com,[10] Figure 3.4 represents another way to look at the normal distribution. It shows the dispersion of values (standard deviations) and what they mean in terms of the percentage of the distribution represented by them.

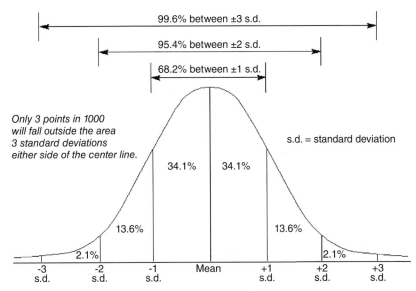

Figure 3.4 Standard deviations from the mean as a function of percentage of distribution.

For example, if your sample mean is 20 and your standard deviation is 2, 68.2% of your values fall between 18 and 22, 95.4% of your values fall between 16 and 24, and 99.6% of your values fall between 14 and 26. This is only relevant if your data are normally distributed, i.e., perfectly centered around the mean.

3.5   The Normal Curve

You can say that a distribution is **normally distributed** because of the shape of the curve being perfectly centered at the mean, which is the equivalent or similar to the median and the mode and is not skewed in one direction or another. It gets a little more complicated, but this curve *represents* the probability (y-axis) or likelihood that a weight value, for example, will be inside the curve in the randomly selected sample, as predicted by your sample weights. Remember that you are approximating weight in your sample as an estimate of all weights in the universe. Since you are setting P (otherwise known as α) at 0.05, this means that 5% of your sample values are in or beyond the two tails of the curve (the shaded region) by chance alone, while 95% of your sample readings will fall within the upper and lower bounds of the confidence interval.

3.6   Sample Size and Power

There are important considerations to take into account when calculating
sample size and **power**:

1. What is your research objective and alternative hypothesis? What is
   your null hypothesis?
2. What is your outcome variable, e.g., cancer remission at 5 years?
3. What is your desired level of power and significance? (How confident
   do you want to be that your sample size will show the hypothesized
   magnitude of sensitivity or specificity with statistical significance or
   disease prevalence, for example?)
4. What is the effect size or quantitative magnitude you have hypothesized? For example, is it 99% sensitivity and 98% specificity, or a 30%
   difference in standardized optical assay readings between two assays, for
   example?
5. What is a scientifically/clinically important effect size?
6. How many patients or samples with the characteristic of interest can
   you produce in your clinic over what period of time, especially if you are
   enrolling patients with rare diseases?
7. What are your cost and time limitations?
8. What about a study dropout rate? If you have a 5% dropout rate
   factored into your analysis, you will need to enroll 5% more patients
   to make up this loss.

The sample size and power to be used in the experiment must be
considered when designing a study, unless you are conducting a pilot study
that provides an estimate of the quantitative parameters in the population.

If you conduct an experiment and find that your experimental test gives
low sensitivity or specificity as compared to a reference test (Sections 8.1.1
and 8.1.2), do you conclude that the test performance is poor? Many would
accept this conclusion. However, did you consider the number of samples
you tested to determine true sensitivity or specificity, for example? Did you
include enough samples to truly determine this level of sensitivity and
specificity in the population?

Calculating sample size and power are essential steps you must take if you
expect to draw meaningful conclusions and publish your results. You may
calculate one or the other; for example, if you have a finite number of patients

that come through a clinic with a particular disease, say 200 patients, then you must limit your sample size to 200 patients and calculate how much power that sample size will offer. However, if you have an infinite number of patients available, then you can set your power at 90%, for example, and see how many patients you must draw from that patient population to satisfy that level of power.

Alternatively, if you are designing a prospective study, and you desire to show differences or equivalency between two samples with a pre-selected power of, say, 80% or better, you would calculate the necessary sample size to show differences or equivalency between two samples.

A word of caution: When calculating sample size and power for performance indicators of a diagnostic test (sensitivity, specificity, positive predictive value, negative predictive value), prevalence becomes an important consideration if you will be evaluating this test in the field. More on these concepts will be discussed in Chapter 8.

Too often, researchers have approached statisticians with the singular question, "how many samples do I need for my study?" without providing details.

As shown in Figure 3.5, there are many ways to calculate sample size or to determine the "power" you have with a set number of samples to make a conclusion. The equation used to determine this depends entirely on the *type* of analysis applied to address your specific aim. In your analysis, you need to consider whether to use a comparison of two means, the establishment of one proportion in a population (e.g., prevalence), a time to death (or other outcome) analysis, a repeated measures ANOVA analysis (analysis of variance), an odds ratio, or a correlation, to mention a few. There are separate sample size equations for each type of primary analysis, and you must determine your objective before selecting a method.

Thus, you could consider using an online sample size calculator to calculate the required sample size based on your objective. Some are more sophisticated than others but if doing simple size and power calculations, try the free **WebPower** download,[11] where you can "crunch" your numbers and also chat with others who post their own questions and advice.

But before we get into the weeds of sample size and power calculations, let's explain a few concepts that are common to all of these calculations.

Type I error: Rejecting a true null finding.
Type II error: Not rejecting a false null finding.

See Figure 3.6 for a graphical representation of Type I and Type II errors.

WebPower Main Menu

Power analysis through Monte Carlo simulation
- Diagram based power analysis (Manual)

Correlation
- Correlation based on Z-test

Proportion
- One sample proportion
- Two sample proportion, equal sample size
- Two sample proportion, unequal sample size

Mean
- Power of t-test
- Power of unbalanced two-sample t-test
- Testing mean with non-normal data (Monte Carlo method)
- One-way ANOVA
- Two-way and three-way ANOVA with interaction
- Repeated-measures ANOVA
- One-way Analogous ANOVA with Binary Data
- One-way Analogous ANOVA with Count Data

Regression
- Linear regression
- Logistic regression
- Poisson regression

Mediation analysis
- Simple mediation analysis based on the Sobel test

Multilevel modeling
- Two level cluster randomized trials with 2 arms
- Two level cluster randomized trials with 3 arms
- Two level multisite randomized trials with 2 arms
- Two level multisite randomized trials with 3 arms

Longitudinal data analysis
- Power analysis for a mixed model of repeated measures with a general correlation structure
- Power analysis for a mixed model of repeated measures with AR(1) correlation structure
- Power analysis for univariate latent change score models
- Power analysis for bivariate latent change score models

Structural equation modeling
- Power analysis based on RMSEA (MacCallum et al., 1996)
- Power analysis using Satorra & Saris (1985)

Figure 3.5 WebPower main menu.

		Truth	
		H_0 **True**	H_0 **False**
Findings	H_0 **True**	Correct	Type II Error (β)
	H_0 **False**	Type I Error (α)	Correct

Figure 3.6 Type I and Type II errors.

Alpha or α: The probability of committing a Type I error which is usually set at 0.05, or 5%. This is also known as the level of significance at or below which you would accept a statistically significant finding. Alpha can also be set at the more stringent 0.025 or 0.01. In addition, the **significance level** (or α) is typically set at 0.05, which is the level at which we would reject the null hypothesis; see Section 3.2.

Beta or β: The probability of committing a Type II error. The acceptable rate of acceptance is around 20% or 0.2, but can be set at the more stringent 10% or 5%.

Confidence interval: $= 1 - \alpha$, or $1 -$ the probability of committing a Type I error, which, with the corresponding level of α, is usually set at 99%, 98%, or 95%.

Power or $(1 - \beta)$: The power is the probability that the test, in this case, will reject a false designation of test inaccuracy, or a false null finding. Of course, one would want to set this level to be high, say 80% or greater, so that it will reject a false designation of test inaccuracy. As power is increased, and therefore precision is increased, the required sample size would increase accordingly. A power of 80% is customarily chosen because most investigators consider that level to be a reasonable level of precision; however, percentage power can be set at a higher or lower level depending on how much error you are willing to accept.

Effect size: When comparing two means for non-equivalency, the difference between the two means is the effect size. When determining a single sample proportion, such as the prevalence of a disease or the proportion of true positives, i.e., sensitivity, your hypothesis is that the prevalence is 3.3%, for example. That is, you are testing that the prevalence in your sample is the same as that drawn from a random population and from previous reported figures, the expected prevalence is 3.3%. The null hypothesis may be that your prevalence is 0%, in which case the effect size is 3.3% – 0% = 3.3%.

To determine effect size, you need to provide the quantifiable associations which are best derived from the literature or from a pilot sample study like we did above to find the 3.3% difference in hypothesized prevalence, i.e., effect size.

More examples of effect sizes are:

- The difference (effect size) in sensitivity between two assays is 6%; sensitivities are 90% and 84%.

- The correlation (effect size) (r) between weight and height is 0.8.
- Patients with poorly controlled diabetes have significantly higher levels of HbA1c (8.5% $\pm$ 2.2%) compared to those with well-controlled diabetes (6.7% $\pm$ 1.2%), effect size is 8.5 – 6.7 = 1.8.

The sample size is the number of samples you will need to test your "alternative" hypothesis against the null hypothesis. It is derived by calculating the number of samples needed to detect an expected effect size as described above, while reducing the possibility of accepting false results. Sample sizes must be based on the primary and/or secondary aims of your study, as described in Section 3.3.

Although it is not shown, the sample size will also increase when the standard deviation of the values in the sample is larger because there is more variability in the data. Producing variation in a carefully controlled experiment can be somewhat reduced, however, when sampling from a homogeneous population or by repeating the experiment in a very controlled manner.

Let's take, for example, motor function testing on five groups: infants, children, young adults, adults, and the elderly. We are quantifying their degree of motor function using the **Wolf Motor Function Test**,[12] which contains 17 questions. Each question is scored from 0 (no ability to perform motor task) to 5 (normal ability to perform motor task), making the total possible range of 0 (unable to perform any of the tasks) to 85 (completes all tasks normally). How many participants would I need to include if I tested the infants, children, young adults, adults, and elderly? I would expect that infants and the elderly may be the least able to complete the tasks, followed by children, and then the adults and young adults may score similarly. This scenario presents a lot of variation and therefore, in order to capture all of this natural variation in all groups, I would need to test a lot of participants. However, if I only tested a more homogeneous group, of young adults and adults, I hypothesize that this variation (standard deviation) would be much smaller (more homogeneous) and I would therefore need to test fewer participants.

Figure 3.7 below shows how sample size, power, and the effect size are all functions of each other and are related. As the effect size (d) increases, the sample size requirement (x-axis) decreases and the power increases. As the effect size gets smaller, the sample size increases and power decreases.

If you want to show equivalence or "non-inferiority" (i.e., no difference) between two assays, your sample size must increase accordingly since you are trying to detect a smaller difference, which after much sampling will require a very large sample size to show this miniscule difference. This is presented in the examples below.

Example for the Epidemiologist

Suppose you wanted to determine the prevalence of the Zika virus in neighboring countries to some of the more heavily impacted regions in Brazil where it is reported to be 0.15–0.66%, according to the Pan American Health Organization (PAHO)/World Health Organization (WHO) Health Emergencies Department (www .paho.org/). Bolivia, for example, lies at the western boundary of these central Brazilian regions. How many samples would you need to test to obtain the true prevalence of the Zika virus in Bolivia?

First, you must determine your null hypothesis. For example, there is no Zika in Bolivia so the prevalence is 0%.

A small study suggested that the prevalence might be close to 1%, so we use that value as the alternative hypothesis. The prevalence of Zika infection in Bolivia is 1%.

The **effect size** will therefore be 1%.

Alternative hypothesis – null hypothesis, or effect size = 1% prevalence – 0% prevalence = 1% .

Okay. How many people in Bolivia do we need to test for Zika virus to assess the prevalence of 1%?

Using WebPower, select "One-sample Proportion" (Figure 3.7) and enter sample size numbers until the calculated power, in the output box, reaches 0.80 or greater.

Given this very small effect size of 1%, you will need to test 85,000 persons to give a true estimate that the prevalence of Zika virus in Bolivia is indeed 1% at 80% power (or certainty).

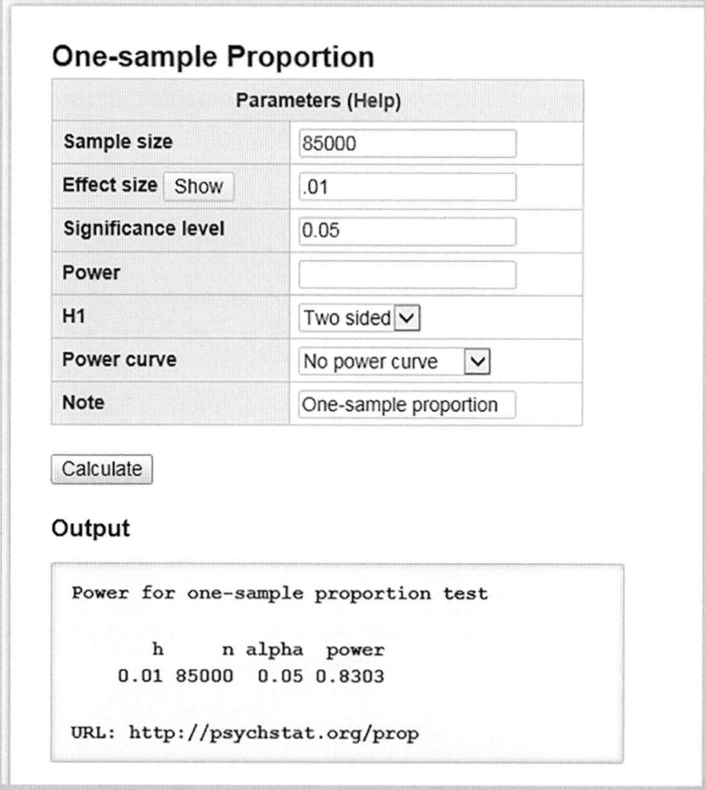

One-sample Proportion

Parameters (Help)	
Sample size	85000
Effect size Show	.01
Significance level	0.05
Power	
H1	Two sided ▾
Power curve	No power curve ▾
Note	One-sample proportion

Calculate

Output

```
Power for one-sample proportion test

      h      n alpha  power
   0.01 85000  0.05 0.8303

URL: http://psychstat.org/prop
```

Figure 3.7 WebPower sample size: Zika.

However, after the fact, suppose after all of this testing, you actually find that the prevalence is much higher than you expected, say 3%, so the effect size now is 3% − 0% = 3%.

Using the same calculator, you can see (Figure 3.8) that you would only need to test 10,000 persons to determine a prevalence of 3%.

So, you have wasted a large number of test kits and substantial technician time because you did not have good evidence from that pilot study, to know what the expected prevalence might be. That is why it is imperative to find other worthy studies in the literature, or to

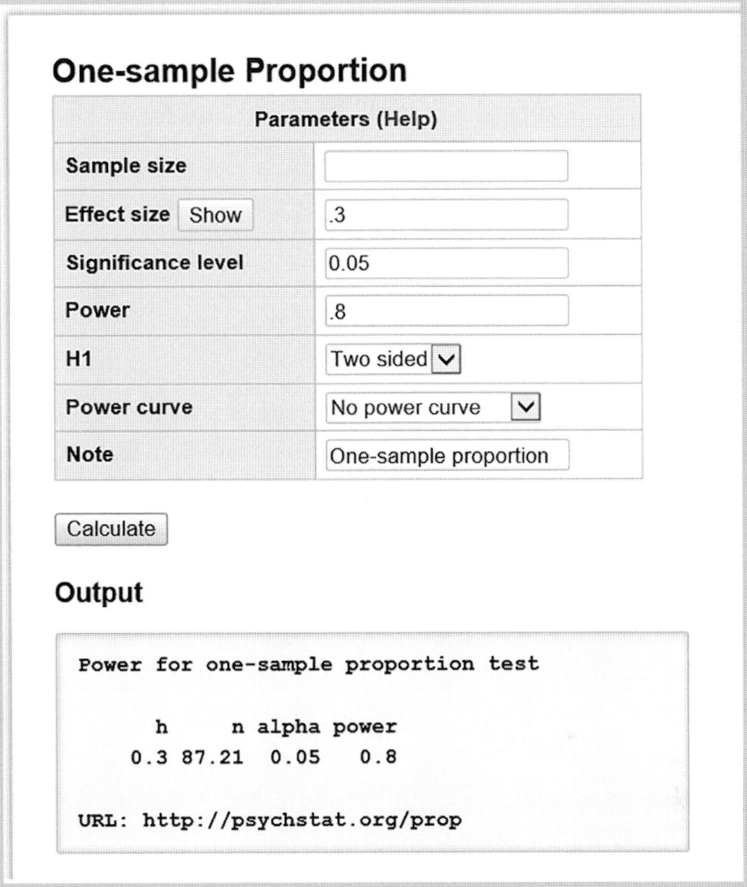

One-sample Proportion

Parameters (Help)	
Sample size	
Effect size Show	.3
Significance level	0.05
Power	.8
H1	Two sided ▾
Power curve	No power curve ▾
Note	One-sample proportion

Calculate

Output

```
Power for one-sample proportion test

     h     n alpha power
   0.3 87.21  0.05   0.8


URL: http://psychstat.org/prop
```

Figure 3.8 WebPower prevalence of 3%.

conduct a pilot study yourself to estimate the prevalence. The Centers for Disease Control (CDC) is also a good source for such information on prevalence and incidence of diseases.[13]

Example for the Clinician

We would like to run a double-blind, placebo-controlled drug trial that examines the efficacy of the standard of care, Drug A vs. Drug A plus the experimental Drug B, and measure the decrease in HbA1c levels on patients with and without well-controlled diabetes. From the animal studies of Drug A and Drug B, and in combination, we have discerned that the addition of Drug B will decrease HbA1c levels by 1.8%.

> *Alternative hypothesis*: Patients on Drugs A and B will have significantly lower levels of HbA1c (6.7% ± 1.2%) compared to those on Drug A alone (8.5% ± 2.2%).
>
> *Null hypothesis*: The HbA1c levels for patients on Drugs A and B will be equivalent to those on Drug A alone, i.e., both will be 8.5% ± 2.2%.

(i)   Choose the **primary analysis** (in this case, a Student T-test of two independent samples is most appropriate; see Section 4.3.1).

(ii) Set up the power calculation as a comparison of two means from two independent samples, i.e., they are in no way related. The T-test is the test used to test for the difference between two means. For example, enter the two means and standard deviations, in this example they are 8.5 ± 2.2 and 6.7 ± 1.2. Although the program will calculate power, enter a power level of 80% in order to solve for sample size.

(iii) From the calculations: sample size will be calculated at the specified power of 80%.

The program will calculate the effect size between the two means and will output the following summary statements (from SPSS Sample Power, Chicago, IL, Release 3.0.1):

- One goal of the proposed study is to test the null hypothesis that the two population means are equal. . . i.e., no difference in HbA1c levels between the two groups.
- The criterion for significance (α) has been set at 0.05. Based on animal studies, the test is set at one-tailed, which means that the experimental drug will decrease HbA1c levels and not increase them, meaning that the effect will be in one direction.
- With the proposed sample size of 17 and 17 for the two groups, the study will have a power of 81.9% to yield a statistically significant result (or difference in HbA1c levels between the two groups). This

computation assumes that the mean difference, or effect size, is 1.8 (corresponding to means of 8.5 versus 6.7) and the common within-group standard deviation (SD) is 1.8 (based on SD estimates of 2.2 and 1.2).

- This effect was selected as the smallest effect that would be important to detect, in the sense that any smaller effect would not be of clinical or substantive significance. It is also assumed that this effect size is reasonable, in the sense that an effect of this magnitude could be anticipated in this field of research.

Of course if you wanted to increase your confidence and precision in these estimates, you may increase your sample size to 20 or 25 patients per group; however, if you decide to test 100 patients but you already detected this difference in the means after testing 25 samples, you can be assured that you have expended some wasteful effort because you detected the hypothesized effect after sampling just 25 patients per group. This is why it is important to meet with a statistician at the very beginning of the study planning process.

Another consideration is where to set levels of acceptance or rejection of Type I error (or α). In this case, we will set α at 5%, that means you will consider your test to be acceptable in comparison to the reference, if the test exhibits an error rate of 5% or less. If you wish to set more stringent bounds on accuracy, as might be requested by the CDC or WHO before test distribution, you may set α to the more stringent 2.5% or 1% error depending on your goal.

Example for the Laboratorian

How many samples do I need to determine if the observed sensitivity of a test is consistent with what the manufacturer claims as the sensitivity of the test?

Alternative hypothesis: 80% of results using Test A would accurately identify positive samples when tested against a "gold standard" test, as stated by the manufacturer of the test.

Null hypothesis: Test A possesses an accuracy rate of ≤80%.

So, what is the effect size? Alternate hypothesis 80%/null hypothesis 70% (choosing one value less than 80) or 10%.

Go to WebPower:[14] bookmark and choose New Analysis → One sample proportion (Figure 3.9).

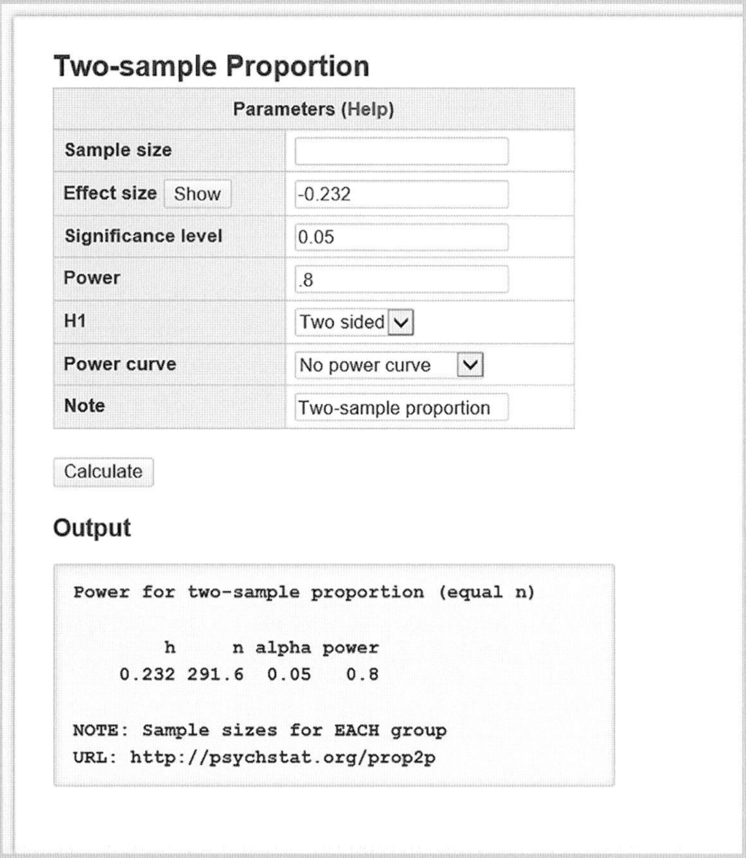

Two-sample Proportion

Parameters (Help)	
Sample size	
Effect size Show	-0.232
Significance level	0.05
Power	.8
H1	Two sided ⌄
Power curve	No power curve ⌄
Note	Two-sample proportion

Calculate

Output

```
Power for two-sample proportion (equal n)

        h      n alpha power
    0.232 291.6  0.05   0.8

NOTE: Sample sizes for EACH group
URL: http://psychstat.org/prop2p
```

Figure 3.9 Sample size between two tests 80%.

- Clear the "Sample size" entry, since that is what you need to calculate.
- In "Effect size, Show," enter 0.7 and 0.8.
- Enter the customary level of "Power at 0.8.
- Press "Calculate" (see Figure 3.10).

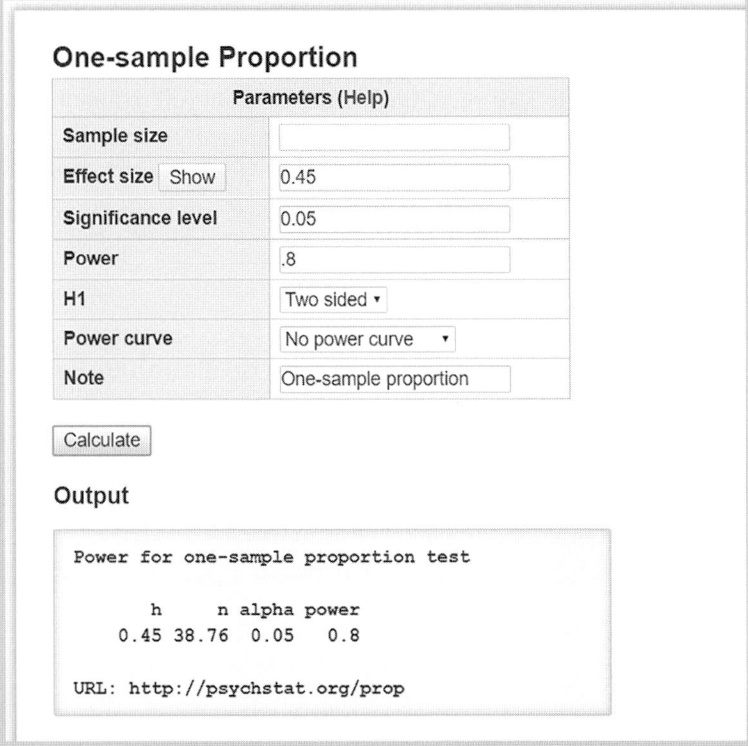

One-sample Proportion

Parameters (Help)	
Sample size	
Effect size Show	0.45
Significance level	0.05
Power	.8
H1	Two sided ▾
Power curve	No power curve ▾
Note	One-sample proportion

Calculate

Output

```
Power for one-sample proportion test

        h      n alpha power
     0.45 38.76  0.05   0.8

URL: http://psychstat.org/prop
```

Figure 3.10 Calculate sample size for a single proportion.

Result: The sample size needed to show this magnitude difference in the proportion of false negatives is $n = 291.6$, or 292 samples.

Regardless of the statistical method on which your sample size calculation is based, you may start your study by calculating sample size at predetermined levels of power and effect size, or you may calculate power at predetermined levels of power and number of subjects or samples. These approaches depend on whether or not you have infinite populations from which to draw samples, or if you have a limited pool from which to draw your samples; if infinite, calculate sample size at 80% or more power; if limited, calculate power setting n at the number of available subjects.

Oftentimes, a statistician will be asked to calculate power and sample size when the effect size is unknown. In this case, the statistician will usually enter a range of clinically reasonable effect sizes. This will give the clinician either a green flag to start recruiting, or the clinician will rethink his study if he cannot possibly recruit the number of needed participants, or one may add recruitment sites to reach the required number. This multi-site recruitment modality is especially common when studying rare diseases, such as Maple Syrup Urine Disease (MSUD).

Sample Size Calculation to Detect a Correlation Between Two Variables (Pearson Correlation Coefficient *r* of 0.6 Between Height and Weight)

Using a **Pearson correlation** for normally distributed data: let's go back to WebPower and begin a new analysis.

New Analysis → Correlation based on Z-test (for normally distributed data)

- Since you are solving for sample size, leave "Sample size" blank.
- We consider a correlation coefficient of 0.4 or greater to indicate a good correlation.
- Since we expect the association of height and weight to be pretty strong, enter 0.6 as the correlation.
- Set significance level at 0.05.
- Set power at 0.8, two-sided, and power curve or no power curve.
- Then click "Calculate."
- WebPower then produces results showing that the sample size of 18.43, or 19 measurements for weight and height, is needed to substantiate this level of correlation, as shown in Figure 3.11. If the hypothesized correlation is higher, i.e., the effect size is larger, you would need fewer cases. You will see; enter 0.8 as the correlation coefficient.

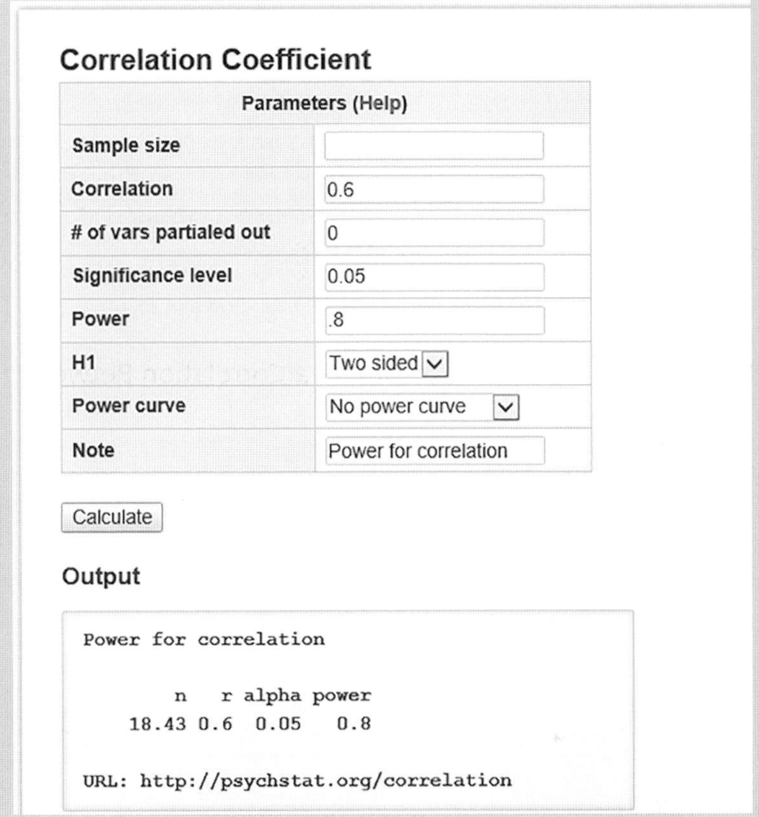

Correlation Coefficient

Parameters (Help)	
Sample size	
Correlation	0.6
# of vars partialed out	0
Significance level	0.05
Power	.8
H1	Two sided ⌄
Power curve	No power curve ⌄
Note	Power for correlation

Calculate

Output

```
Power for correlation

        n    r alpha power
    18.43 0.6  0.05   0.8

URL: http://psychstat.org/correlation
```

Figure 3.11 Calculate sample size to test for a correlation.

Sample Size Calculation to Detect One Proportion

The prevalence of Atrial Septal Defect (ASD) and Ventricular Septal Defect (VSD) among Downs Syndrome patients in the US is 10%. We want to know if we are finding similar rates of ASD and VSD in Europe. How many Downs Syndrome patients with coronary heart disease (CHD) should I screen to find the true prevalence of ASD and VSD in Europe?

Go back to WebPower → New Analysis → One proportion:

- Leave sample size blank.
- Effect size is 0.1 (=10%).
- Set power at 0.8.
- Two-sided.
- Then "Calculate."

To detect a prevalence of ASD and VSD of 10%, one would need to sample 784 persons with Downs Syndrome and CHD, as shown in Figure 3.12.

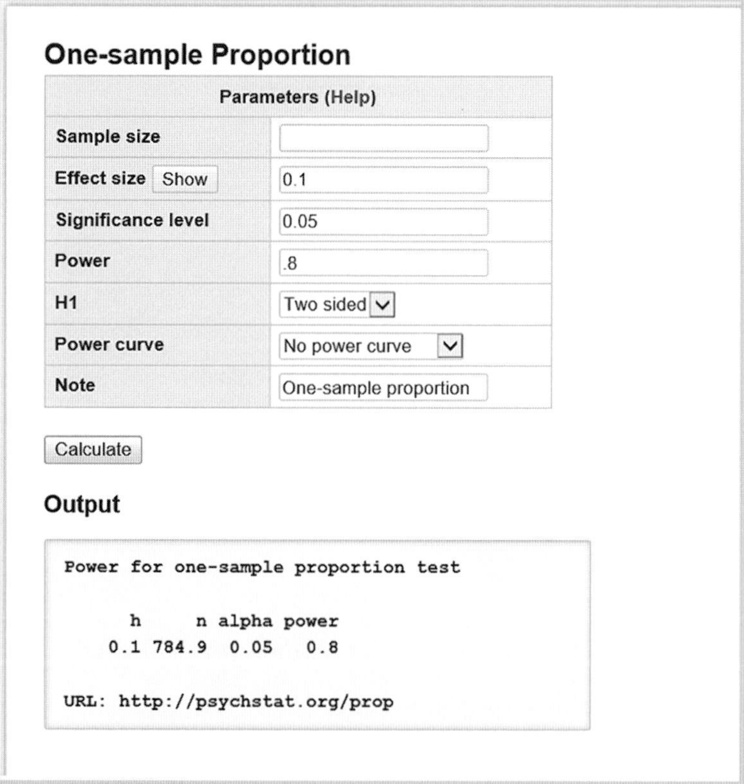

One-sample Proportion

Parameters (Help)	
Sample size	
Effect size Show	0.1
Significance level	0.05
Power	.8
H1	Two sided ✓
Power curve	No power curve ✓
Note	One-sample proportion

Calculate

Output

```
Power for one-sample proportion test

     h     n alpha power
   0.1 784.9  0.05   0.8


URL: http://psychstat.org/prop
```

Figure 3.12 Calculate sample size to test for a prevalence of 10%.

So, now we have learned some basic concepts about power and sample size. As stated earlier, these concepts range much beyond what is mentioned here, as they are also applied to many other study designs which take on other considerations and calculations. It would be wise to consult with a statistician when methodologically and statistically designing your study and setting up your sample size calculations, particularly if you are applying for research funding. Keeping that statistician on board throughout your research project would also be beneficial to the efficiency of study continuation.

Links to Online Tools

[10] Syque.com
[11] https://webpower.psychstat.org/wiki/
[12] http://dx.doi.org/10.13072/midss.257
[13] www.cdc.gov/datastatistics/index.html
[14] https://webpower.psychstat.org/wiki/models/index

II The Right Statistical Test for Different Types of Data

4 Analyzing Continuous Data

Well, what kind of data do you have?

This chapter focuses on guidance in selecting the appropriate statistical test depending on what type of data is being analyzed. Remember, data can be continuous, binary, ordinal, nominal, normally distributed, non-normally distributed, log-distributed, and so on (Chapter 2). Decisions must be based on a full understanding of the kind of data you have and your analytic objective. Conduct your preliminary analyses! Plot your data! Look at your data! Do you have outliers, skewness, errors?

4.1 Single Continuous Distribution

Univariate analyses are used to explore single variables at a time. Types of univariate data analyses are:

- mean (Section 1.5.1)
- mode (Section 1.5.3)
- range (Section 1.5.4)
- interquartile range (Section 1.5.5)
- skewness (Section 1.5.6)
- kurtosis (Section 1.5.7)
- frequency distributions (Section 1.6).

These are just a few of the ways you can describe a single variable. Examples of these univariate statistics are available in Sections 1.5 through 1.7.

4.2   Visual Comparison of Two Continuous Variables Using Scatterplots

Although not a statistical test, one important first step in visualizing your bivariate continuous data is in the form of **scatterplots** (see Chapter 10).

Scatterplots, which may easily be performed in Excel, can provide a clear snapshot of whether or not variables are associated or completely disassociated, such as weight vs. height, rain in inches vs. plant growth. When drawing a tight-fitting line through the scatter dots, meaning a line from which the dots are best fitted, a good correlation is one where the distance of the dots from the line is minimal (see Section 4.3.3 for more on correlations).

In another example, plotting the results of Test A against Test B (Figure 4.1) shows that the values are linearly related, but their scales of increase vary on the x- and y-axes. So, before you decide that they are perfectly linear, be sure to look at the rates of rise on the y-axis and run on the x-axis. This visual determination will not necessarily confirm their

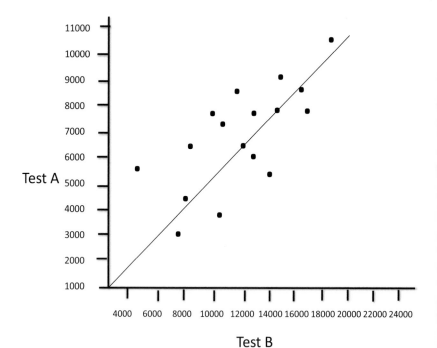

Figure 4.1 Typical scatterplot.

associations; we have other statistical tests for that, but viewing scatterplots can give a fairly good estimate of associations between two continuous variables.

4.3   Two or More Continuous Distributions

There are two types of analyses to use when comparing two continuous distributions: (a) testing relationships of one continuous variable between two groups, or (b) comparing two dependent, continuous variables to each other. Depending on how the continuous variables are distributed, you would need to select different statistical techniques as described below.

In both of these circumstances, we are conducting a **bivariate analysis**, which refers to the analysis of two variables, in this case, distributions of continuous variables at the same time, whether it is between two independent groups or between two independent variables. The comparison can be between two groups of specimens or persons that are unrelated or independent (data not from the same specimens or persons), or can be between two dependent, continuous values, such as the correlation of height vs. weight from the same persons.

4.3.1   *T*-test

Normally distributed, continuous data from two independent samples can be analyzed using a *T*-test. A **T-test** is a bivariate test that compares means and variances of data from two independent groups, that is, from groups that are not related in any way, such as the comparison of height between boys and girls. Before considering running a *T*-test on data, be certain that the distributions are normally distributed for both groups by (a) comparing the mean to the median to be sure that they are approximately equivalent (see Section 1.5) and (b) conducting frequency distributions for each group, plotting normal curves over the data points to visually see if the data conform to the normal distribution. When data from both groups have been confirmed as being normally distributed (Figure 4.2), an independent samples *T*-test can be performed to compare mean weight between boys and girls, for example. (If they are not normally distributed, proceed to Chapter 5.)

(a)

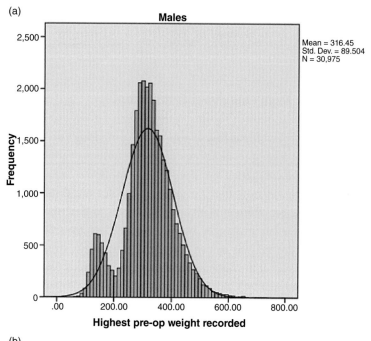

(b)

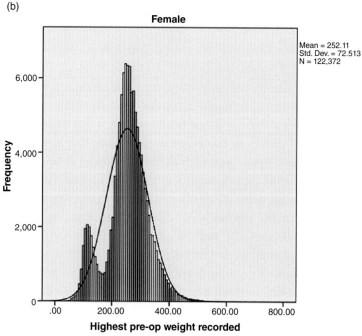

Figure 4.2 Weight distribution for (a) boys and (b) girls.

Table 4.1 T-test of pre-operative weight before bariatric procedure

T-test

	Sex	N	Mean weight (lbs)	Std. dev.	Std. error mean
Pre-op weight closest to bariatric surgery	Male	33,812	269.6383	102.82912	0.55922
	Female	134,281	216.1588	83.65013	0.22828

Independent samples test

	Levene's test for equality of variances	T-test for equality of means			95% CI of the difference	
	Sig.	d.f.	Sig. (2-tailed)	Mean difference	Lower	Upper
Pre-op weight closest to bariatric surgery	Equal variances assumed	0.000	168,091	0.080	53.47950	52.43189	54.52711
	Equal variances not assumed		45,698.269	0.000	53.47950	52.29562	54.66338

Although these do have bimodal distributions, i.e., they have two peaks in the distribution, we can assume, for now, that both of these distributions are approximately normal.

The *T*-test compares not only the means between two groups, but also the variation of the two distributions of two independent samples (see Table 4.1). The *T*-test generates two sets of *P*-values: one for the difference between the means and another for the difference between the variances (or standard deviations), called Levene's test for equality of variances. So, before deciding which *P*-value for mean differences to report, look at the Levene's test *P*-value. If it is less than 0.05, you can firmly state that equal variances are not assumed (i.e., standard deviations are not equal) and you must, therefore, report the two-tailed significance of $P = 0.001$. Had you assumed that the variances were equal, you may have incorrectly reported that the mean difference is not statistically different at $P = 0.08$.

The numeric results in Table 4.1 show that males have a significantly higher pre-operative weight than females, but what *P*-value do I state? You can see that Levene's test for equal variances shows that $P < 0.001$, meaning that the variances (standard deviations 102.83 and 83.65) are statistically different (as denoted by the Levene's *P* of 0.000), so the proper *P*-value associated with the significance of the whole *T*-test is that standing with unequal variances, which is 0.000 (or better stated, <0.001).

As stated previously, you can set your *P*-value, meaning that you will accept significance at ≤ 0.05 or ≤ 0.01 or ≤ 0.001, depending on the certainty one wishes to set. However, when *P*-values are displayed in tables, such as the one in Table 4.1, 0.001 is actually the calculated value for *P*. If you set your level of certainty at $P < 0.001$, you may reject significance at the calculated value of *P*.

Let's try one on our own. Suppose you have two groups of women, one group is pre-menopausal and the other is post-menopausal. We want to compare estrogen levels between these two groups.

- Go to www.socscistatistics.com/tests/studentttest/default2.aspx *T*-test calculator for two independent means and look at Figure 4.3(a). Notice that the calculator appears to be set up to compare the effects of two treatments. One can simply consider these as the two independent groups of data.

(a)

The Friedman Test for Repeated Measures

The Kolmogorov-Smirnov Test of Normality

Kruskal-Wallis Test Calculator for Independent Measures

Levene's Test of Homogeneity of Variance Calculator

Mann-Whitney U Test Calculator

Sign Test Calculator

Standard Error Calculator

T-Test Calculator for 2 Independent Means

T-Test Calculator for 2 Dependent Means

T-Test Calculator for a Single Sample

Wilcoxon Signed-Rank Test Calculator

Z Score Calculator for a Single Raw Value

Z-Test Calculator for a Single Sample

Z-Test Calculator for 2 Population Proportions

Figure 4.3 Example of using a free, online, *T*-test calculator.

- I will enter the estrogen levels (in pg/mL) for one group in Treatment 1 and the other group in Treatment 2 (Figure 4.3b).
- I will then set my significance level at 0.05 and select a one-tailed test since it is well documented that post-menopausal women will have significantly lower estrogen levels, so the effect can only go in one direction.
- Then, press "Calculate T and P Values."

So, without getting into the import of the *T*-value, let's just say that the difference between pre-menopausal and post-menopausal estrogen levels is significantly different at $P < 0.000088$, as shown in Figure 4.3(c).

(b)

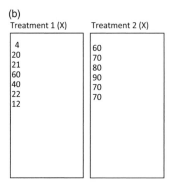

Treatment 1 (X)	Treatment 2 (X)
4	60
20	70
21	80
60	90
40	70
22	70
12	

(c)

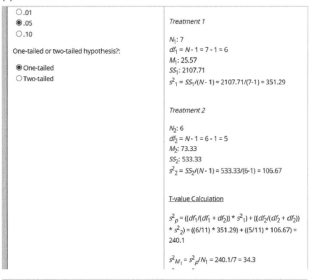

○ .01
◉ .05
○ .10

One-tailed or two-tailed hypothesis?:

◉ One-tailed
○ Two-tailed

Treatment 1

N_1: 7
$df_1 = N - 1 = 7 - 1 = 6$
M_1: 25.57
SS_1: 2107.71
$s^2_1 = SS_1/(N - 1) = 2107.71/(7-1) = 351.29$

Treatment 2

N_2: 6
$df_2 = N - 1 = 6 - 1 = 5$
M_2: 73.33
SS_2: 533.33
$s^2_2 = SS_2/(N - 1) = 533.33/(6-1) = 106.67$

T-value Calculation

$s^2_p = ((df_1/(df_1 + df_2)) * s^2_1) + ((df_2/(df_2 + df_2))$
$* s^2_2) = ((6/11) * 351.29) + ((5/11) * 106.67) =$
240.1

$s^2_{M_1} = s^2_p/N_1 = 240.1/7 = 34.3$

$t = (M_1 - M_2)/\sqrt{(s^2_{M_1} + s^2_{M_2})} = -47.76/\sqrt{74.32} = -5.54$

The t-value is -5.54042. The p-value is .000088. The result is significant at $p < .05$.

Note: If you wish to calculate the effect size, this calculator will do the job.

Want to know how to report this t-test result in your work? (Opens in a new tab so you don't lose your calculation.)

How to report a t-test result (APA)

Calculate T and P Values   Reset

Figure 4.3 (cont.)

Table 4.2   Example of an ANOVA procedure

	Treatment days from dx.				95% CI for mean		
	N	**Mean**	**Std. dev.**	**Std. error**	**Lower bound**	**Upper bound**	**P-value**
Region 1.00	295,830	25.27	32.321	0.059	25.15	25.38	
Region 2.00	290,899	25.14	31.642	0.059	25.03	25.26	
Region 3.00	318,359	23.05	31.692	0.056	22.94	23.16	<0.001
Region 4.00	199,027	22.60	29.242	0.066	22.47	22.73	
Region 5.00	220,029	26.25	32.697	0.070	26.11	26.39	
Total	**1,324,144**	**24.47**	**31.667**	**0.028**	**24.41**	**24.52**	

4.3.2   ANOVA

Remember, the null hypothesis, when comparing means (review Section 3.3) assumes that all means and standard deviations are equal. The alternative hypothesis is that the means and standard deviations are significantly different. The analysis of this variance gives the ANOVA its name, because it is a tool used precisely to compare means and standard deviations across three or more independent and unrelated groups, such as shown in Table 4.2. It's a good tool to use to visualize multiple means and standard deviations but it doesn't tell you what group is statistically different from the other. In Table 4.2, you might consult the 95% confidence intervals to see which intervals are overlapping, which means that the groups are not statistically different, or if they are not overlapping, meaning that they are statistically different.

Also, when comparing three or more groups on a continuously and normally distributed variable, one can apply an ANOVA. Again, the only drawback when comparing three or more groups, such as "Number of Treatment Days," for example (Table 4.2), is that when you look at the results of an ANOVA you don't know what group is statistically different from the other. You just know that all together, the mean number of days from diagnosis to treatment is significantly different between all regions. In order to know what regions are truly different, one would have to group, say, regions 3 and 4 (the lower values) and regions 1, 2, and 5 (the higher values) and run a T-test. However, this can sometimes lead to situations where you are conducting multiple T-tests, so if you get above 20 *T*-tests, you may need to apply the Bonferroni correction (Section 3.1), lowering the threshold of acceptance at $P < 0.01$.

You can run your ANOVA using an online calculator.[15]

4.3.3   Pearson Correlation

A **Pearson correlation**, which compares the linear relationship between two variables, is the appropriate test to use for continuous and normally distributed variables, such as height vs. weight.

The Pearson correlation coefficient (r) ranges from -1 to 1 (see Figure 4.4).

- $r = 1$ when there is a perfect, positive correlation, such as height vs. weight, where they both vary in the same positive direction.
- $r = -1$ when there is a perfect, inverse relationship between two variables, like the amount of water consumed and the degree of dehydration, where they both vary in the same negative direction.
- $r = 0$ when there is a flat-line relationship between two variables, like the height of Maryland residents and the number of light bulbs in houses in Maryland, i.e., no relationship, although, beware of attempts to show spurious correlations between bizarre characteristics such as height and the number of light bulbs!

A Pearson correlation measures the linearity between two continuous and normally distributed variables; thus, it is another example of a parametric analysis. In general, you can state that variables are considered to be positively correlated if $r \geq 0.4$ or inversely correlated if $r \leq -0.4$, however, it really depends on what variables are being compared and their biological relationship. I wouldn't expect height and weight to correlate less than 0.7 unless you are analyzing data on obese patients, for example, where r might be around 0.5 because weight is proportionally higher and less tightly associated with height.

So, when we run the Pearson correlation statistic (Figure 4.4 and Table 4.3), we see that $r = 0.587$, which is a pretty strong correlation coefficient of weight vs. height. The two-sided significance is 0.000, so it is statistically associated. However, it is the magnitude and the direction of the correlation that are more

Table 4.3   Example of a Pearson correlation

Baseline height		Baseline weight
	Pearson correlation (*r*)	**0.587**
	Sig. (2-tailed)	0.000
	N	6863

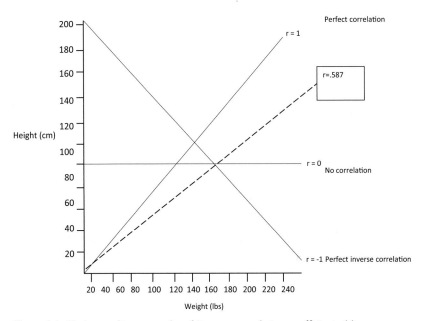

Figure 4.4. Understanding strengths of Pearson correlation coefficients (*r*).

important than statistical significance. The two-sided *P*-value is used in this example as we allow the effect to be in two directions, i.e., height and weight of individuals could be positively correlated or inversely correlated. However, in other systems, such as determining the correlation of a test assay against a gold-standard assay, you will want a much higher, positive correlation, say *r* = 0.95–1.0. It is a clinical and laboratory judgment call when accepting that two variables are, or are not, associated.

One concept that cannot be overstated about Pearson correlations is the dispersion of the association. It is possible that results from a standard cell

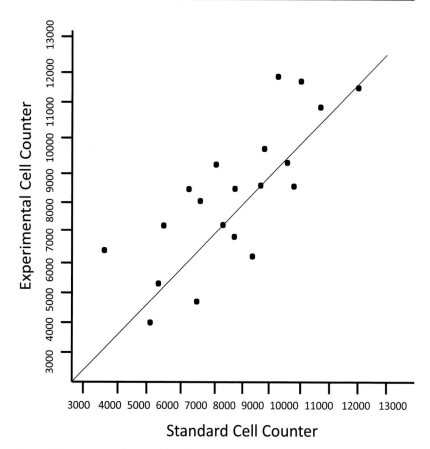

Figure 4.5 Depiction of a correlation between two cell counters.

counter-correlate well with the results of a gold-standard cell counter, for example, where many results may stray from the correlation line, as shown in Figure 4.5.

So, if you draw a line through the data points of the scatterplot, it becomes evident, from Figure 4.5, that the experimental cell counter is almost perfectly correlated with the standard, or the correlation gives an r value above 0.9, for example, but there is some deviation from that correlation line. This deviation leads one to use another statistical approach that considers the "scatter" from the correlation line, the **regression analysis**, which is discussed in Section 7.3.2.

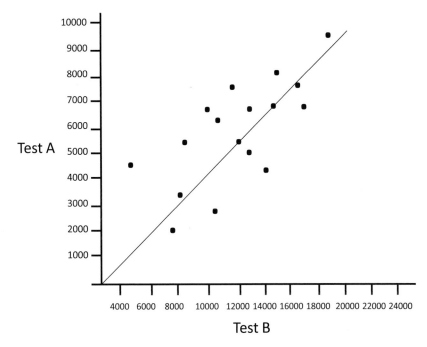

Figure 4.6 Correlation between two tests.

Another consideration about Pearson correlations is the scale of increase in both variables. Suppose you are measuring the equivalence of two laboratory assays by applying a Pearson correlation technique. You may find a strong correlation between the test values (i.e., $r \geq 0.8$, for example), but the values in Test B rise at nearly twice the rate of those in Test A, so they definitely are not equivalent. If they were equivalent, the rise and run on the x- and y-axes would be the same: with every 1-point rise in Test A, there is a 1-point rise in Test B. Notice the incremental increases on the x-axis of Figure 4.6, which are nearly twice that of the y-axis (Figure 4.6). In other words, two variables can be highly correlated but not equivalent. Be sure to study your data using graphical techniques like the scatterplot, before drawing conclusions about their associations.

If you choose not to perform the Pearson correlation calculation in Excel, and you want to calculate it manually, you can construct a table like Table 4.4. The expression for r is as follows:

Table 4.4 Example of how to manually calculate a Pearson correlation

Record	Weight (x)	Height (y)	xy	x^2	y^2
1	100	60	6000	1000	3600
2	50	30	1500	2500	900
3	80	40	3200	6400	1600
Total ($\sum$)	$\sum x = 230$	$\sum y = 130$	$\sum xy = 10{,}700$	$\sum x^2 = 9900$	$\sum y^2 = 6100$

$$r = \frac{N\sum xy - (\sum x)(\sum y)}{\sqrt{\left[N\sum x^2 - (\sum x)^2\right]\left[N\sum y^2 - (\sum y)^2\right]}}$$

where

N = number of pairs of scores

$\sum xy$ = sum of the products of paired scores

$\sum x$ = sum of x scores

$\sum y$ = sum of y scores

$\sum x^2$ = sum of squared x scores

$\sum y^2$ = sum of squared y scores

But I promised no equations! See the Pearson correlation calculator.[16] Now it's just a matter of entering the column totals into the equation, but usually you are analyzing more than three records at once so making a mistake would be much more probable. If you need to satisfy your curiosity in understanding this calculation further, there is more information at the same calculator and you can run your own Pearson correlation.

4.4   Two Normally Distributed, Continuous Distributions from Samples that are Related

Now we have a situation where we have one normally distributed, continuous variable measured twice on the same person or on the same specimen.

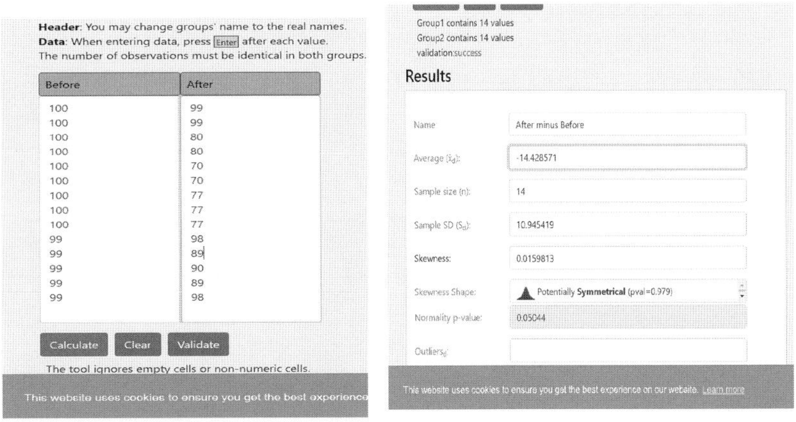

Figure 4.7 Free online paired *T*-test (StatsKingdom.com).

Let's go to the psychometrics lab for this one. In this case, we would use a tool that is similar to the *T*-test, but instead of being based on the difference between the means and variances of two independent distributions, we are looking at paired differences within subjects or within samples, and the distribution of those differences along a continuum. For obvious reasons, it is called the paired *T*-test and it is applied to paired situations, as shown in Figure 4.7.

Example for the Clinician

I am measuring the intelligence quotient (IQ) in 15 teens before and after partaking in cannabis consumption with the hypothesis that their IQ scores before consumption are significantly higher than their IQ scores after consumption. Notice in this example that the number of teens is fixed, while the level of power floats and is completely influenced by *N*. With 15 paired measurements, I have 80% power to detect an average of a 20% decline in IQ. I did not select 80% power; that is what an *N* of 15 paired observations calculated for me.

I will collect the pre-consumption IQ scores, then collect the post-consumption IQs (see Figure 4.7). Let's go to StatsKingdom to enter our results and run the program.[17] Then enter the pre- and post-consumption IQ data directly into the tables provided.

Voila! My hypothesis is correct again! How we wish science were this perfect! Cannabis consumption results in significantly reduced IQ points, averaging a 4-point loss after one round of consumption, $P = 0.0057$ (as shown in Figure 4.8).

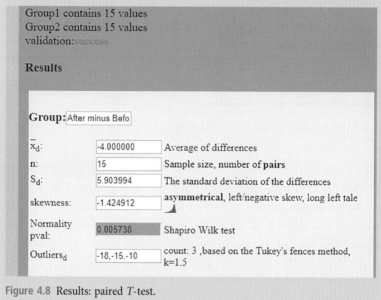

Group1 contains 15 values
Group2 contains 15 values
validation: success

Results

Group:	After minus Befo	
$\bar{x}_d$:	-4.000000	Average of differences
n:	15	Sample size, number of **pairs**
S_d:	5.903994	The standard deviation of the differences
skewness:	-1.424912	asymmetrical, left/negative skew, long left tale
Normality pval:	0.005738	Shapiro Wilk test
Outliers$_d$	-18,-15,-10	count: 3 ,based on the Tukey's fences method, k=1.5

Figure 4.8 Results: paired *T*-test.

Please keep in mind that these are not actual statistics from actual studies, but are merely created for teaching purposes.

Example for the Laboratorian

In the laboratory, we would like to test cell viability at baseline and after 70 days of being slowly frozen in glycerol at $-80°C$. Our hypothesis is that the cells will lose at least 20% of their viability; my null hypothesis is that they will not lose any viability. After running a sample size calculation,[18] I found that 15 specimens on which we will make these paired comparisons will give me 83% power to show this 20% decline. In this example, I let the program determine the power of the analysis instead of setting power at a certain percentage. The data collection was performed in StatsKingdom (Figure 4.9).[19] This time,

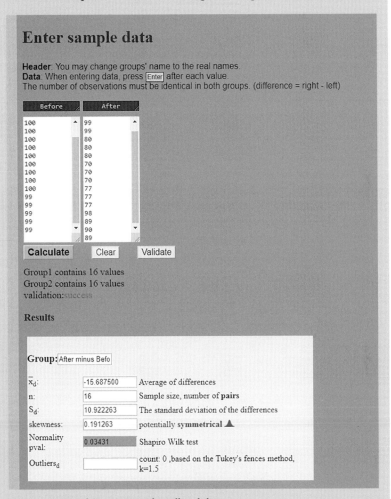

Figure 4.9 Paired *T*-test example: cell viability.

I will set the test to calculate significance at a one-tailed value. Why? We know the cells cannot increase their viability above 100%, and the literature tells us that viability will decline in such conditions, so we only expect one direction of change, i.e., a reduction, if at all.

So, we find that the average decline in viability in our cells as a product of freezing is 15.7%, which is significant at a one-tailed *P*-value of 0.034.

Links to Online Tools

[15] https://goodcalculators.com/one-way-anova-calculator/

[16] www.socscistatistics.com/tests/pearson/Default2.aspx

[17] www.statskingdom.com/160MeanT2pair.html

[18] www.sample-size.net/sample-size-study-paired-t-test/

[19] www.statskingdom.com/160MeanT2pair.html

5 Analyzing Non-normally Distributed, Continuous Data: Non-parametric Tests

Again, parametric procedures are preferred over non-parametric because parametric analyses are more robust in that they use the actual values of the distribution in the analysis. If the data are incapable of becoming "normalized" by transforming the distribution to approximate a normal distribution, such as taking $\log_{10}$ of all HIV viral load values, non-parametric tests should be applied to examine your data. Let's examine some non-parametric approaches to analyzing non-normally distributed data. In general, two tests, the Mann–Whitney U test and Spearman rank test, fall into this analytic category. In short, the Mann–Whitney U test is the non-parametric equivalent to the T-test and the Spearman rank test is the non-parametric equivalent to the Pearson correlation.

5.1 Mann–Whitney U Test (aka Wilcoxon Rank Sum Test) of Two Independent Samples

Let's assume you have run frequency distributions on all your data and have attempted to superimpose a normal curve on some variables and have examined the skewness only to find that your data are not normally distributed (review Chapter 6) and are incapable of being transformed to approximate a normal distribution. When the median is far from the mean and attempts to transform the data to normality have failed, it would be appropriate to apply a non-parametric procedure to compare the distributions of these values in two samples. One way to achieve this is by using a procedure called the Mann–Whitney U test.

Like the parametric T-test, the **Mann–Whitney U test** is the non-parametric equivalent that tests for significant differences between non-normally distributed, continuous variables. Because ordinal variables have a non-quantitative but ordered distribution, the Mann–Whitney U test can also be used to test for differences between ordinal distributions. Like the T-test, the samples must be independent (i.e., not from the same or related persons or samples). These tests are based on ranking each value from lowest to highest for all values (both groups), so the actual values will lose their numerical identity, so to speak, which is why we consider parametric procedures to be more robust. However, sometimes, we have no choice on which set of procedures to use. So, as the values are ordered, each receive a rank score that expresses each value's position in the distribution.

Example for the Laboratorian

Suppose we are running a cell viability study using two different cell media; we want to determine if the new test medium is any better than the standard medium.

Null hypothesis: The new test medium is no different than the standard medium in terms of supporting cell viability.
Alternative hypothesis: The new test medium is better than the standard medium in terms of supporting cell viability (thus, a one-sided hypothesis!).

Remember that the higher the viability of cells, the better the medium in supporting their viability, so keep this directionality of the results in mind when accepting or rejecting your hypothesis.

Notice in Table 5.1 that two of the viability values are the same (82%), so it would be wrong to give them different rank scores of 4 and 5 because numerically, they are the same. The way to give them equal weight is to give each the mean of 4 and 5, which is 4.5.

Table 5.1   Manual calculation of a Mann–Whitney U test

	Cell viability	
	Standard media (rank)	**Test media (rank)**
	83% (6)	92% (8)
	82% (4.5)	70% (3)
	68% (2)	90% (7)
	52% (1)	82% (4.5)
Sum of ranks	$R_1 = 13.5$	$R_2 = 22.5$

So, 92% loses its identity by becoming a rank of 8, and 52% becomes a rank of 1; you can see how the actual percentage viability values become almost insignificant. More important is where they rank amongst themselves. Thus, this may better convince you that running parametric statistics with actual values gets us closer to the truth and is much easier to interpret. Therefore, we do all that we can to "normalize" the data (if possible) rather than having to resort to non-parametric methods.

Normally, you will have many more records so, although it would be somewhat unwieldy to calculate manually, you can run this test in a statistical analysis program or in Excel by using the `rank.avg` function for all of the scores. Then, calculate the sum of ranks using the `sumif` function (identify data range).[20]

So, by going back to the sample media and cell viability example, the Mann–Whitney U test statistic is calculated for two samples (standard vs. test media) as:

$$U_1 = n_1 n_2 + \frac{n_1(n_1 + 1)}{2} - R_1;$$

$$U_2 = n_1 n_2 + \frac{n_2(n_2 + 1)}{2} - R_2.$$

Here, U_1 and U_2 are the Mann–Whitney U test statistics, n_1 and n_2 are the sample sizes of the standard and test media, respectively, and R_1 and R_2 are the sums of the ranks for standard and test media, respectively:

standard n_1 = 4
new test n_2 = 4
standard R_1 = 13.5
new test R_2 = 22.5.

Now, just enter the numbers:

Standard media $U_1 = 4(4) + \dfrac{4(4+1)}{2} - 13.5 = 16 + \dfrac{20}{2} - 13.5 = 16 + 10 - 13.5 = 12.5.$

New test media $U_2 = 4(4) + \dfrac{4(4+1)}{2} - 22.5 = 16 + \dfrac{20}{2} - 22.5 = 16 + 10 - 22.5 = 3.5.$

In this particular experiment, the number of readings for both media is 4, so the first part of the calculation $[n_1 n_2 + n_1(n_1 + 1)]$ is a constant in the calculations of U_1 and U_2. However, in the real world, most experiments can result in one or more invalid or missing readings and, thus, result in unbalanced sample sizes; so, in addition to the different U_x, the n values would also impact these calculations.

In this example we find that U_2 is lower than U_1, which supports the research hypothesis that the new test medium is better than the standard medium in supporting cell viability. Why is a lower score better? Well, let's think how the scores were derived. Lower U scores mean that the sum of ranks for the test medium (R_2) was larger, meaning that they contributed to higher cell viability. This larger R is then subtracted from the rest of the quantity, making the resulting U score lower (review the equation again). So, the sum of the ranks for the test medium (R_2) is larger than the sum of the ranks for the standard medium (R_1), resulting in a lower U score.

Obtaining a P-value for the Mann–Whitney U test requires consulting a complicated table, and that gets into probably more than you want to know, so the best recommendation is that you use a program that will do this for you.[21] In the output, you can see that a "critical value" of U is mentioned. This is a value that is selected from a Mann–Whitney U table by cross-referencing sample size 1 and sample size 2 and finding that critical value in the table.

5.2   Spearman Rank or Spearman's Rho Coefficient (Independent Observations)

To examine the correlation between continuous data from two samples, we rely on the Pearson correlation analysis or its non-parametric equivalent, the Spearman rank coefficient. Recall that when we examined the relationship between weight and height, we applied a Pearson correlation. Why? Because the distributions of weight and height were normally distributed. However, if one or more variables is not normally distributed, we must use ranking procedures, much like we did in the Mann–Whitney U test.

Example for the Clinician

Suppose you were planning to conduct a study to discern if an increase in emergency department (ED) support staff might reduce the time (in minutes) to fully process an ED patient through all necessary procedures or to hospital admission.

Alternative hypothesis: An increase in support staff will significantly reduce ED patient processing time.

Null hypothesis: An increase in support staff will not reduce ED patient processing staff.

Method: In a controlled manner, we will increase ED support staff by one person every three days (to account for between-day variation) and measure average, daily patient processing time (in minutes) over the course of 21, 10-hour shifts and collect the data in Figure 5.1(a).

Results: Your resulting data are distributed as such. You might say that ED staff numbers are normally distributed, but clearly processing minutes are not, as shown in Figure 5.1(b). In this case, a Spearman rank correlation test would be appropriate to test for an association between the two.

(a)

Day	Number ED staff	Patient processing (minutes)
1	4	25.00
2	4	30.00
3	4	40.00
4	5	40.00
5	5	32.00
6	5	19.00
7	6	25.00
8	6	19.00
9	6	30.00
10	7	21.00
11	7	22.00
12	7	21.00
13	8	18.00
14	8	35.00
15	8	40.00
16	9	20.00
17	9	17.00
18	9	16.00
19	10	17.00
20	10	20.00
21	10	16.00

Figure 5.1 Correlation analysis of non-normally distributed data: (a) data table; (b) frequency plot.

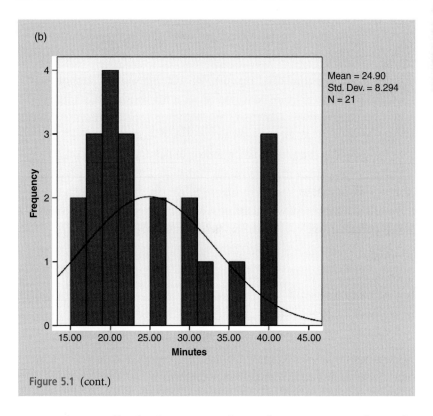

Figure 5.1 (cont.)

Mathematically, the Spearman rank correlation is very similar to the Mann–Whitney U test where one calculates each value's distance from the median, so I won't go through the step-by-step calculations again, but I will introduce you to the Spearman rho calculator.[22] By copying and entering your x-values (minutes) and your y-values (number of staff) into the table (or entering the values directly into the application), you should come up with a Spearman rank, $r_s = -0.62744$, P (2-tailed) = 0.00233, meaning that we see a significant inverse correlation ($r_s = -0.62744$), i.e., an increase in support staff correlates with a significant ($P = 0.0023$) decrease in patient processing, thus proving that the alternative hypothesis is correct! Don't you wish all process-improvement endeavors could be so successful?

Links to Online Tools

[20] https://www.youtube.com/watch?v=pwZuo4bc-GE
[21] http://www.socscistatistics.com/tests/mannwhitney/Default2.aspx
[22] https://www.socscistatistics.com/tests/spearman/Default2.aspx

6 Analyses for Non-continuous Data

6.1 Binary Data

Some examples of binary data (or **dichotomous data**) are:

- yes/no
- true/false
- reactive/non-reactive
- 0 = no disease/1 = disease
- 0 = test negative/1 = test positive, etc.

Sometimes these variables are also called **qualitative data**, since they do not specify quantities (as quantitative data do).

So, if we compare two binary variables (e.g., gender by disease/no disease), you might construct a contingency table that looks like Table 6.1.

6.1.1 Contingency Tables and Chi-Square Test

A **contingency table** is a table that shows the distribution of one variable within categories of another, like gender vs. disease/no disease. These tables can be 2×2, 2×3, 2×4 (if you were to examine gender by race, for example), 2×6, etc. The second variable can have two values (such as yes or no) or three or more values like race (White, African American, Asian, etc.). When examining a 2×2 table like disease by gender, one would test for statistical significance using chi-square (χ^2) analysis. However, like ANOVA (Section 4.3.2), when including a variable that has more than two categories, like race, you can run the χ^2 statistic but there are so many resulting cells, you won't really know where the statistical differences lie since you are examining so many categories at once.

Table 6.1 Comparison of two binary variables – contingency table

	Disease	No disease	Total
Male	10	20	**30**
Female	2	28	**30**
Total	**12**	**48**	**60**

Chi-square measures for differences between the observed number of observations minus the expected number of observations. So, what are the observed and expected numbers?

Let's say that Laboratory 1 and Laboratory 2 are counting the number of test kits that are defective in the lot that they each received.

Alternative hypothesis: Lab 1 received significantly more defective test kits than Lab 2.

Null hypothesis: There is no difference in the proportion of defective kits in Lab 1 and Lab 2.

We can set the significance at $P \leq 0.05$. The first thing we do is construct a contingency table by entering the observed values, as shown below. Beside the observed values in parentheses are the cell labels as an assist.

	Lab 1	Lab 2	Total
Not defective	70	10	80 **(A)**
Defective	50	20	70 **(B)**
Total	120 **(C)**	30 **(D)**	150 **(A+B)**

Now we need to calculate the expected values. The expected numbers come from the null hypothesis, i.e., if there is no difference in the delivery of defective kits for Laboratories 1 and 2, then all **proportions** of defective kits over the total number of delivered kits to both labs should be equal, right? Wrong. Since the labs received different numbers of kits, we just have to calculate the expected numbers by hand. Notice the bolded cell designations above, the numbers of which are to be entered into the following equations to calculate:

$\dfrac{A \times C}{A + B}$	$\dfrac{A \times D}{A + B}$
$\dfrac{C \times B}{A + B}$	$\dfrac{B \times D}{A + B}$

$$\text{Expected A} = \frac{80 \times 120}{150} = \frac{9600}{150} = 64.$$

$$\text{Expected B} = \frac{80 \times 30}{150} = \frac{2400}{150} = 16.$$

$$\text{Expected C} = \frac{120 \times 70}{150} = \frac{8400}{150} = 56.$$

$$\text{Expected D} = \frac{70 \times 30}{150} = \frac{2100}{150} = 14.$$

Now, applying the chi-square formula where O = observed and E = expected:

$$\chi^2 = \sum \frac{(O - E)^2}{E}.$$

In English:
chi-square = sum of (observed values – expected values) squared, divided by the expected value.
   So:

$$\chi^2 = \frac{(70 - 64)^2}{64} + \frac{(10 - 16)^2}{16} + \frac{(50 - 56)^2}{56} + \frac{(20 - 14)^2}{14}$$
$$= 0.56 + 2.25 + 0.64 + 2.57 = 6.02.$$

Mapping this χ^2 value of 6.02 with a P-value becomes a bit difficult and since it is unlikely that one will calculate these values by hand, this discussion will be discontinued at this point.

We complete the example above on the chi-square calculator[23] by first entering the category titles, then "Next," then entering the original values into the cells of the table. Set the significance at the desired level, then calculate chi-square; the *P*-value is 0.01409, which is highly significant and confirms the alternative hypothesis that Lab 1 received a significantly higher proportion of defective test kits than Lab 2.

Notice, though, that when you see the 2×2 table as shown for Lab 1 and Lab 2, it might appear that you are performing a non-parametric analysis, since the outcome variable is binary, i.e., defective = 1/non-defective = 0. However, note that it is actually a parametric analysis because the observed minus expected generates a continuous distribution of numbers, i.e., 0.56, 2.25, 0.64, 2.57, which is shown towards the bottom of the example above. So, by constructing a 2×2 table, or a $2 \times n$ table, you can quickly appreciate the simplicity of the analysis at hand.

Example for the Clinician

Are the rates of a disease more prominent in males or females? That's easy: among males, there are 10/30 (or 33.3%) with the disease, while in females, there are 2/30 (or 6.67%) with the disease. But are these dissimilar rates clinically significant? They certainly appear to be.

But are they statistically and significantly different? How do we make this 2×2 comparison? The best way to compare these two rates is by using the chi-square analysis.

Alternative hypothesis (based on your research on the topic): The prevalence rates of disease are at least 5 times higher in males than in females.

Null hypothesis: the prevalence rates of disease are the same in males and females.

- How many samples do you need to make this comparison with adequate precision and power?
- We actually only need 10 males and 10 females to achieve 86% power to detect this effect size of 5 times higher, for example 1% vs. 5%. But to increase precision (see Section 3.6), we tested 30 of each gender.

So, rather than calculating the chi-square manually, we use a simple online chi-square calculator.[24] Following Figure 6.1, enter your numbers in the tool, and then click "Next."

Chi-Square Calculator

The next stage is to fill in your data. Remember, the data is categorical - the number of subjects observed for each cell.

Enter Your Data Below						
	Disease	No Disease				
Males	10	20				
Female	2	28				

Please enter your categorical data, then press Next.

Next

Figure 6.1 Free online chi-square calculator.

Set your significance level (usually 0.05), but if you are running many multiples of exploratory chi-square tests, consider applying the Bonferroni correction (Section 3.1) and accept significance at the more stringent 0.01. Click "Calculate Chi^2," then you receive your result (Figure 6.2).

Results						
	Disease	No Disease				Row Totals
Males	10 (6.00) [2.67]	20 (24.00) [0.67]				30
Female	2 (6.00) [2.67]	28 (24.00) [0.67]				30
Column Totals	12	48				60 (Grand Total)

The chi-square statistic is 6.6667. The p-value is .009823. The result is significant at $p < .05$.

Start Again

Figure 6.2 Chi-square calculator results.

When you have small sample sizes, i.e., when one of the cell entries is five observations or less, the **Fisher's exact chi-square** statistic gives a better approximation of significance than the chi-square statistic. Thus, given the small sample size, one should cite the Fisher's exact statistic of 0.0211 in this example, which is significant at $P < 0.05$. The Fisher's exact or the chi-square may be used for large sample sizes, but it must be used in small sample sizes. The tool to use for the Fisher exact test can be found online.[25]

6.1.2   Odds Ratios, Risk, and Relative Risk

Using the same example, what are the **odds** of getting the disease for males and for females? Using the same tool, as shown in Figure 6.3,[26] you may actually calculate the odds of the disease as well as the risk and relative risk of the disease by gender (1 = males, 2 = females). Note that we are no longer using the chi-square or the Fisher's exact statistic, although they appear similar in the way we set them up.

- **Risk** – the probability of a disease or, for example, the number with the disease in males divided by the number of males.
- **Relative risk** – for males, the probability of a disease occurring in males divided by the probability of it occurring in females, and vice versa for calculating the relative risk for females. The calculations are shown below.
- **Odds ratio** – the odds that an outcome, like a disease, will occur in response to a given exposure, compared to the odds of it occurring in the absence of the exposure.

		Result			
	Bad Outcome	Good Outcome	Total	Risk	Odds
Group 1	10	20	30	0.33	0.5
Group 2	2	28	30	0.07	0.07
Total	12	48			

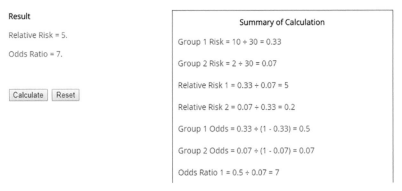

Result

Relative Risk = 5.

Odds Ratio = 7.

Calculate   Reset

Summary of Calculation

Group 1 Risk = 10 ÷ 30 = 0.33

Group 2 Risk = 2 ÷ 30 = 0.07

Relative Risk 1 = 0.33 ÷ 0.07 = 5

Relative Risk 2 = 0.07 ÷ 0.33 = 0.2

Group 1 Odds = 0.33 ÷ (1 - 0.33) = 0.5

Group 2 Odds = 0.07 ÷ (1 - 0.07) = 0.07

Odds Ratio 1 = 0.5 ÷ 0.07 = 7

Figure 6.3 Free online calculator of odds ratios, risk, and relative risk.

Table 6.2 Calculation of odds ratio

	Disease	No disease	Total
Exposure	10 a	20 b	30
Non-exposure	2 c	28 d	30
Total	12	48	60

Looking at Table 6.2, for example, the odds ratio for those who were exposed to a teratogen is ad/bc = $10 \times 28/20 \times 2 = 280/40 = 7$. That is, those who were exposed to cigarette smoke, for example, have 7 times the odds of developing lung cancer. If the odds ratio is 1, that means there is no significant increase or decrease in the odds of developing the disease due to the exposure; "those who were exposed have 1 times the odds of developing the disease...," which means no increase.

Likewise, if the 95% confidence interval of the odds ratio crosses 1, the exposure is said to have no impact on the development of disease.

Another way to calculate the odds ratio is by performing what is called a **binary logistic regression** (which will be discussed in Section 7.1).

6.1.3   Kappa Statistic

A **Kappa statistic** is a measure of agreement between two raters on a binary measure, positive/negative, etc. It is also a measure of interrater reliability or interrater agreement.

Let's take a simple clinical example.

Let's say that two radiologists were independently reading (rating) X-ray films to determine their interrater agreement on detecting wrist stress fractures. The shaded boxes in Table 6.3 show the number of films that they agreed were indeed stress fractures ($n = 10$) and which ones were not ($n = 2$). So, you might think that the level of agreement is $\frac{(10 + 2)}{19} = 0.63$, right? Well, no, that's not right, but that IS the observed agreement.

Table 6.3   Calculation of the Kappa statistic

		Rater 2	
		Fracture +	Fracture −
Rater 1	Fracture +	10(A)	4(B)
	Fracture −	3(C)	2(D)

Now we must take into account that the raters might not be able to definitively determine if the stress fracture is present or absent, so they will use some method of equally balancing their judgments on both sides of the fracture diagnosis. This we term a random answer. So, they may randomly say yes, fracture or no, no fracture because they are not certain how to rate it. We must account for this randomness in our Kappa calculation. Note that this may not seem intuitive; this is an example of "just do it as instructed" and you will get the right answer!

The probability of agreement is

Pr = probability

$$Pr_{agreement} = (A + B/A + B + C + D)*(A + C/A + B + C + D)$$

$$Pr_{non\text{-}agreement} = (C + D/A + B + C + D)*(B + D/A + B + C + D)$$

Now, let's just work through the math.

$$Pr_{agreement} = (10 + 4/19) \times (10 + 3/19)$$
$$= 14/19 \times 13/19 = .73 \times .68 = .4964$$

$$Pr_{non\text{-}agreement} = (3 + 2/19 \times 4 + 2/19)$$
$$= 5/19 \times 6/19 = .05 \times .31 = .5199$$

Now the Kappa statistic, or the level of agreement is $Pr_{agreement} + Pr_{non\text{-}agreement} = .4964 + .0155 = .5199$ (or 52%) which indicates moderate agreement on the scale.

Kappa Agreement Scale

0 = agreement equivalent to chance
0.1–0.2 = slight agreement
0.21–0.4 = fair agreement
0.41–0.6 = moderate agreement
0.61–0.8 = substantial agreement
0.81–0.99 = near perfect agreement
1 = perfect agreement.

It's easy to see how random decisions can impact the level of agreement. This can also be applied to laboratory experiments, to run an assay to determine the interrater reliability of the positive or negative status of specimens. This is an especially useful tool when training residents or laboratory technicians to read films, or assay results, respectively.

So, you can either go through the nuances of calculating Kappa manually, or use a free online calculator.[27]

6.2   Ordinal Data

Ordinal data are "ordered" variables that give a sense of quantity, but the distance between the values cannot be quantitatively measured. For example, what is the quantity between a weak signal and a moderately weak signal? There is none.

So, it would be impossible to use a parametric statistic on ordinal data since the mean of non-quantitative ordinal values is really irrelevant. You would not calculate the mean for the agree to disagree scale, would you? There are no interval markings between values on a Likert scale, so there is no such mean. So, it is best to apply a non-parametric statistic, like the median or mode, when describing the distribution of an ordinal variable.

The **Kruskal–Wallis** test is another non-parametric test that is appropriate to use for ordinal data as it tests for distributional differences between three or more independent groups; it is an extension of the Mann–Whitney U test (Section 5.1) that tests for non-parametric differences between two ordinal distributions (like the ANOVA is to the T-test, the Kruskal–Wallis test is to the Mann–Whitney U test). An online Kruskal–Wallis calculator is available,[28] in which you can enter your ranked values, i.e., 1 (for poor) to 5 (for great).

6.3   Nominal Data

Nominal data, in contrast, are completely non-quantitative, non-interval, and data that may only be included in non-parametric analyses (Section 1.4) such as contingency tables (not chi-square or Fisher's exact tests though), frequency distributions, etc. Nominal variables are usually used as grouping variables on which to compare continuous or non-continuous variables. As an example of how nominal data are used as grouping variables, you may want to conduct an ANOVA analysis that compares age, for example, the mean and SD of CD4 T-cells by race, or CD4 T-cells by HCV vs. HIV vs. HCV + HIV groups.

6.4   Time-to-Event Data

Time to death, time to cell replication, time to disease recurrence, etc. You may have heard of the term "life tables" when discussing the time to a discrete event. A life table is simply a depiction of instances when outcomes occur, e.g., time to death for cancer patients.

6.4.1   Kaplan–Meier

The **Kaplan–Meier** estimate is the most common type of life-table approach to examine the kinetics of patient loss due to death, for example, but can also be used to examine time to any event, like time to cancer remission or time to cell proliferation. Figure 6.4 gives an example of a Kaplan–Meier plot.

The typical data elements required to run a Kaplan–Meier analysis are:

- group (bile spillage = 1, no spillage = 0)
- months surviving (or until death, loss to follow-up, or until end of observation period)
- date of event (if the event occurred)

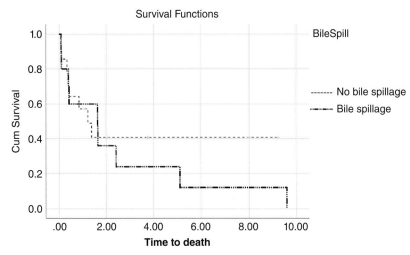

Figure 6.4 Example of a Kaplan–Meier plot.

- calculate time to event = date of event – cohort entry date
- designation of event (1 = event occurred, 0 = event did not occur).

Those who are either lost to follow-up or for whom the event did not occur during the observation period are "censored" from the analysis, meaning that they contribute useful data up until the time of their disappearance from the study sample. Kaplan–Meier plots can be constructed for one study sample or for more than one. In Figure 6.4, you can see a Kaplan–Meier plot (using SPSS V. 22) for gallbladder removal patients who either experienced bile spillage or did not. The survival time starts at 1.0 (or 100% of the sample) and drops vertically when the event (death) occurs, then moves horizontally as time passes. A **log-rank test** is used to compare the survival "curves," which shows that those with bile spillage (median 0.55 months) have a significantly shorter time to death than those without bile spillage (3.74 months), $P = 0.004$.

A tool can be used to run your own Kaplan–Meier for two patient samples, like the one shown above.[29] Denote censored cases by asterisks. It is important to plot the 95% confidence bands as they do show some overlap in the early part of the observation period, meaning that the two groups of patients are declining at approximately equal rates, but then they diverge significantly as time goes on.

6.4.2   Cox Proportional Hazards Model

But like nature, time to death, or to any other event, is influenced by many variables. Stage of cancer, for example, will likely impact time to death, so how do we weave this effect into our time-to-event analysis? We do this by constructing a **Cox proportional hazards model**, where we calculate how much hazard is introduced when one accounts for cancer stage or age or insurance status, all of which can be entered into the model at once. Unfortunately, a coherent online tool for running a Cox proportional hazards model could not be found, so you will need to have a statistician run this analysis for you. Additionally, there are some statistically advanced nuances that may require help from a statistician.

There is another free program that can estimate the required sample sizes and power for both the Kaplan–Meier and the Cox proportional hazards model analyses.[30] It also includes the sample size and power calculations for many other procedures.

Links to Online Tools

[23] https://www.socscistatistics.com/tests/chisquare2/default2.aspx
[24] https://www.socscistatistics.com/tests/chisquare2/default2.aspx
[25] https://www.socscistatistics.com/tests/fisher/default2.aspx
[26] https://www.socscistatistics.com/biostatistics/Default2.aspx
[27] https://www.easycalculation.com/statistics/cohens-kappa-index .php
[28] https://www.socscistatistics.com/tests/kruskal/Default.aspx
[29] http://www.evanmiller.org/ab-testing/survival-curves.html
[30] http://powerandsamplesize.com/Calculators/Test-Time-To-Event-Data/Cox-PH-Equivalence

7 Analyzing a Combination of Data Types When the Outcome is Binary

7.1 Binary Logistic Regression and Calculation of Odds Ratios and 95% Confidence Intervals

One commonly used analytic technique that examines predictors of a binary outcome (disease/no disease, test positive/test negative, etc.) is called a logistic regression. As it is for other types of regression analyses, the final set of predictors that are added to the regression equation must all be present for each case that is included in the final analysis pool. The most important point when building a model is not to enter all variables in a haphazard fashion. There are specific steps to arriving at the final set of predictors.

The steps used to arrive at a set of predictors to enter into a regression equation are as follows:

- Run multiple bivariate analyses with variables of interest against your single, binary outcome variable.
- Select variables that are statistically and significantly different for those with the outcome versus those not with the outcome at $P < 0.05$.
- Select from that set, variables that make clinical sense as a predictor of the outcome; those that make clinical sense as being known to impact the outcome variables, such as gender, weight, age, for example, should be kept in the equation all of the way to reaching the final model. This is known as "while correcting for gender, weight and age, the odds of developing an outcome is..."
- Ensure that there are not conditional variables in the set of predictors, i.e., you would not want to add gender and pregnancy (yes/no) as that would exclude all males since they will all have missing data for their pregnancy status.

- Look for variables that are correlated with each other by running either a Pearson correlation or a Spearman rank correlation, depending on the distributions of the variables.
- If you find that two variables are highly correlated, i.e., $r \geq 0.4$ or $r \geq 0.8$ depending on the variables being correlated, select one variable that has the least non-missing values, so you can optimize the number of cases being included in the binary logistic regression analysis.
- By this point, you should probably have two to six predictors (otherwise known as covariates) to enter into your equation. Why "covariates"? Because together, they co-vary the variation in the outcome variable.
- Enter these variables into the logistic regression tool, run the analysis, and keep only the variables that have $P \leq 0.10$ (remove all others) and run it again, until you have narrowed the list of predictors down to those with the lowest P-values and the highest odds ratios. But why select variables at $P \leq 0.10$ when we usually set P at the tighter constraints of ≤ 0.05 or ≤ 0.01? This is a judgment call when the number of candidate variables are few, thus, loosening the criteria for entry into the logistic regression is practiced.

Use the free online logistic regression calculator[31] and start entering data as directed in Figure 7.1.

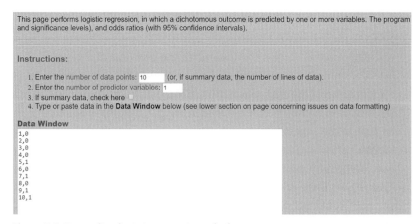

Figure 7.1 Free online logistic regression calculator.

- First, enter the number of records (what they call data points, which is not quite correct), which in this case is 10.
- Then, enter the number of predictors, which in this case is 1. In your data window, the item you enter will be the predictor variable(s) which may be continuous, binary, nominal, or ordinal. In this case, the predictor variable is continuous and ranges from 1 to 10.
- After entering all of your predictor variables, followed by a comma, the last variable you enter is the outcome, like 0 for no disease and 1 for disease.
- Press "Solve."
- As stated above, remove the columns of data (predictor variables) as you hone in on the set of predictors that give the highest odds ratios with 95% confidence intervals that do not cross 1.
- After removing columns of data, solve again.

Keep in mind that your dataset will hopefully have more than 10 records of data. So, you can save your data into a *.csv file (which places commas between the values, making certain that your outcome variable is listed in the last column), then you can copy and paste the contents of your *.csv file into the data window.

As shown in Figure 7.2, the P-value(s) (0.0979 in this case) and the 95% confidence interval (0.8852–4.2478) can be found in the results box.

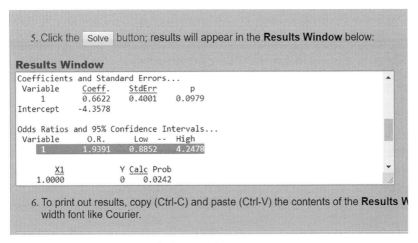

Figure 7.2 Logistic regression calculator results.

Table 7.1 Alternative method to calculate an odds ratio using known indices of disease status and exposure status

Elevated catecholamine?	CHD (disease variable)	
(Exposure variable)	Yes (1)	No (0)
Yes (1)	27	95
No (0)	44	443

Interpretation: This one predictor is not a good predictor of the outcome because the 95% confidence interval crosses 1, which means that the predictor does not predict the outcome. Further, the *P*-value (0.0979) does not meet the set criteria of being ≤ 0.05.

This program can also analyze summary data. For example, Table 7.1 summarizes information on 609 individuals by exposure (catecholamine) and disease (CHD).

Below, two examples of logistic regressions are presented to show how this procedure is applied.

Example #1. Using the data in Table 7.1, the data can be entered as summary data in two lines in the format: exposure variable level (0 and 1), number *without* disease (95 and 443) at this exposure level, number *with* disease at this exposure level (27 and 44).

In this example the number of data points is two, the number of predictor variables is one, and check the "summary data" box. The complete example data are shown below, with the variable being exposure category, number without CHD in exposure category, and number with CHD in exposure category. You could copy these data and paste them in the data window:

1, 95, 27
0, 443, 44

The results of the analysis would be as follows, exactly the same as the "data at the individual level, one exposure variable" example shown previously, based on the same data:

Variable	Odds ratio	95% CI (low–high)
Elevated catecholamine	2.8615	1.6878–4.8514

Table 7.2 Logistic regression output (N = 809,434)

Outcome: 30-day readmission	Predictor step 1 OR (95% CI)			Predictor step 2 OR (95% CI)		
	OR	Lower	Upper	OR	Lower	Upper
Age	1.002	0.974	1.030			
Gender	0.977	0.518	1.841			
Race	0.951	0.793	1.141			
Payer	0.971	0.668	1.412			
Income national quartile	0.859	0.652	1.130			
Holiday	2.744	1.378	5.462	2.367	1.243	4.510
Distance*	0.996	0.991	1.002			

which presents as a strong predictor of CHD. As stated in a manuscript, "Those exposed to catecholamine possess a 2.367 odds of developing CHD (95% CI 1.6878–4.8514) than those who were not exposed."

There is really no need for a P-value here, since the 95% confidence interval, which does not cross 1, explains the significance of its predictive ability to explain the variance in the outcome, CHD from 0 (no CHD) to 1 (CHD).

Example #2. Here is another example of a binary logistic regression (Table 7.2). In step #1, I entered all variables that had independent, bivariate associations with a hospital 30-day readmission. I followed all of the necessary steps to pare down the number of covariates, as described earlier. In this table, you can see that all but one of the covariates (predictors) have 95% confidence intervals that include 1, and therefore are not acceptable predictors of 30-day readmission. The only predictor that stood out was whether or not surgery occurred during the holiday season. Those having surgery during the holiday season had a 2.7 odds of a 30-day hospital readmission, 95% CI 1.24–4.5 than those who had surgery during non-holiday months.

7.2   ROC Analysis

One of the more elegant procedures, although not statistical, is the **receiver operator characteristic (ROC)** curve analysis. It is often used to find cutoffs along a continuum where the sensitivity and specificity of a continuous variable are optimized to stratify on a binary "gold-standard" outcome.

Table 7.3 ROC table of disease status vs. continuous test variable

Gold standard disease status (known disease status) 0 = non-diabetic 1 = diabetic	HbA1c (%)
0	2
0	7
0	7
0	3
0	2
0	3
0	5
0	6
1	7
1	7
1	8
1	5
1	10
1	14
1	5
1	8

Let's use a laboratory example to illustrate. We are developing a test that rapidly identifies diabetics at point-of-care centers in the community such as mobile vans, remote clinics, and at health fairs. Test results are available after 15 minutes and it only uses a small swab of oral fluid from the patient's buccal cavity. After conducting a sample size calculation based on the test's sensitivity to accurately identify those who are positive for diabetes, we must enroll 50 diabetic patients and 50 non-diabetic patients. Their known disease status is determined by a standard test known as the "gold standard."

The test gives quantitative measures of HbA1c level in the saliva and the values range from 2% to 14%.

To find the optimal cutoff that best distinguishes diabetics vs. non-diabetics using my new assay, we will perform the swab test, gather data, and generate Table 7.3 in order to perform a ROC curve.

Now, let's plot a ROC curve. Using the free and downloadable software, PSPP[32] you will see a way to run the ROC analysis and many other procedures. It looks strangely like SPSS, but is a bit more limited in its offerings.

After entering your numbers into the PSPP spreadsheet (Figure 7.3a, b), go to "Analyze, ROC Curve," then enter the test variable (HbA1c), the state variable (which is the gold-standard variable "Diabetes"), and the value of the state variable (which is coded as 1 for a known diabetic). Think of the "state" variable as the disease state, the number that indicates the presence of disease.

Figure 7.3c shows the area under the curve (AUC), which in this case is 0.89. It also shows the ROC curve. If the AOC was 1.0, the test would have perfect sensitivity and perfect specificity, so an AUC of 0.89 is pretty high.

In the plot showing the ROC curve, the star is not produced by this program but has been added to approximate the highest sensitivity and lowest 1-specificities (highest specificity) convergence.

It might seem counter-intuitive to plot sensitivity against 1-specificity. Why don't we just plot sensitivity against specificity? Because if you look at sensitivity on the x-axis and specificity on the y-axis, there is really no visual or quantitative method to select the optimal sensitivity or specificity while optimizing the area under the curve. However, when sensitivity is plotted against 1-specificity, one can easily see the point at which the line peaks closest to the x-axis yet lowest on the y-axis (the star in Figure 7.3c).

These points correspond to an HbA1c value of 6.5, which is where sensitivity and specificity are the optimal cutoffs of this test for discriminating between diabetics and non-diabetics; at a level of 6.5, the test is 83% sensitive and $1 - 0.25 = 0.75$, or 75% specific.

These are not great performance indices. If this were the case, we might develop a second test, using the same oral fluid specimen, that is optimized for maximal specificity. So, for my first test, I can set the test to discriminate diabetics with 86% sensitivity at a HbA1c level of 4.10, which will likely capture a few negatives. To circumvent that problem, the second highly specific test would identify the false positives, so we could reclassify them as non-diabetic with some degree of accuracy.

7.3   Continuous Outcome

7.3.1   Regression Analysis

Regression analysis compares the relationship between one or more variables of any type (continuous, ordinal, nominal, binary) and the outcome (which is continuous). But is it similar to a Pearson correlation?

(a)

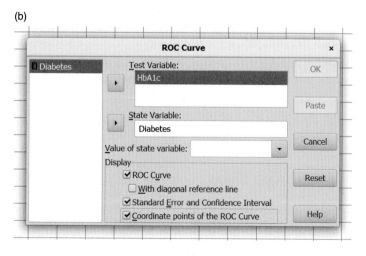

(b)

(a) ROC spreadsheet; (b) enter coordinates; (c) table of coordinates.

Figure 7.3 (a) ROC spreadsheet; (b) enter coordinates; (c) table of coordinates.

(c)

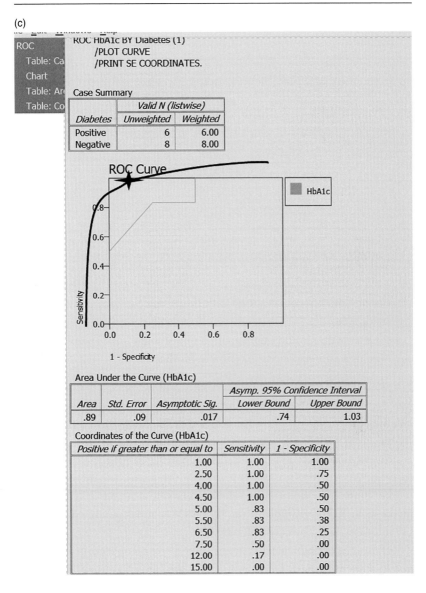

ROC HbA1c BY Diabetes (1)
    /PLOT CURVE
    /PRINT SE COORDINATES.

Case Summary

| Diabetes | Valid N (listwise) | |
	Unweighted	Weighted
Positive	6	6.00
Negative	8	8.00

Area Under the Curve (HbA1c)

| Area | Std. Error | Asymptotic Sig. | Asymp. 95% Confidence Interval | |
			Lower Bound	Upper Bound
.89	.09	.017	.74	1.03

Coordinates of the Curve (HbA1c)

Positive if greater than or equal to	Sensitivity	1 - Specificity
1.00	1.00	1.00
2.50	1.00	.75
4.00	1.00	.50
4.50	1.00	.50
5.00	.83	.50
5.50	.83	.38
6.50	.83	.25
7.50	.50	.00
12.00	.17	.00
15.00	.00	.00

Figure 7.3 (cont.)

While the regression analysis is still a way to explore the linear relationship between two or more variables on an outcome variable, it differs from the Pearson correlation as it also calculates the best-fitting line that describes the data while minimizing the scatter from the line; Pearson

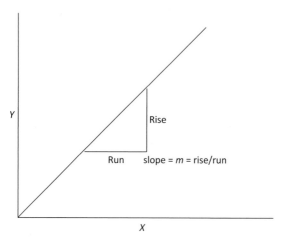

Figure 7.4 Slope of a line.

correlation does not concern itself with the distance of each point from the regression line.

Let's start with recalling the equation of a straight line (Figure 7.4). The equation of a straight line is $Y = mX + b$, where

Y is the value of the variable on the y-axis, and is the dependent variable

X is the value of the variable on the x-axis and is the independent variable

b is the y-intercept (or where the regression line originates on the y-axis)

$$m = \text{slope} = \frac{\text{rise}(Y)}{\text{run}(X)}.$$

The slope of the line can be calculated to find how much X influences increases in Y. For example, it can explain how much saturated fat intake (X) increases LDL cholesterol levels (Y).

But, as in most biological systems, such direct comparisons are usually not so straightforward. Other influences, like lack of exercise, can play a key role in rising LDL levels. To account for the simultaneous impact of exercise and fat intake, this is where we must add "covariates" such as exercise level to the equation:

$$Y = mX + b + \beta x_1$$

where

X is fat intake (in grams)

Table 7.4   Regression output

| Model dependent variable LDL | Unstandardized coefficients | | |
	β coefficient	Std. error	Sig.
1 b (y-intercept)	7.931	0.733	0.000
Fat intake	−0.270	0.126	0.048
Exercise	−1.084	0.757	0.097

Y values are the LDL levels (in mg/dL)

b is the y-intercept (or where it crosses the y-axis)

$$m = \text{slope} = \frac{\text{rise}(Y)}{\text{run}(X)}$$

βx_1 = amount Y changes for a unit increase in x_1 (a covariate).

β is called the **beta coefficient**, otherwise known as the **regression coefficient**.

Let's get back to our example. You may use Excel to run regressions (e.g., the LINEST function) or the other free software PSPP or R. Or, you may use statistical packages such as SAS, SPSS, or STATA.

Let's run an analysis on a small dataset:

Dependent = LDL level (mg/dL)

Predictors: Fat intake (10–100 g/day)

Level of exercise (0 = never exercise to 10 = exercise often).

We run the regression using this one dependent variable, LDL level, and our two hypothesized influencers (predictors) of LDL increase, and get the results shown in Table 7.4.

Remember: $Y = mX + b + \beta x_1$.

So, LDL levels = −0.270 × (fat intake) + 7.931 − 1.084 × (exercise).

Now, we will accept that lack of exercise is a good predictor of increased LDL, despite having a P-value of 0.09. As described earlier, we can accept an association in a regression if the P-value for a predictor (or covariate) is ≤ 0.1 to maximize the number of predictors entered in the regression.

When we enter multiple predictors into a regression equation, the formula becomes

$$CY = mX + b + \beta x_1 + \beta x_2 + \beta x_3 + \beta x_4 + \beta x_5$$

where $\beta x_1 + \beta x_2 + \beta x_3 + \beta x_4 + \beta x_5$ is the product (or multiplier) of the beta coefficient of that predictor and the actual value of that predictor in your dataset, such as 1.084 times the value for exercise in your dataset.

Mathematically speaking, the beta coefficient for these predictors is what I like to call the *weight* of that predictor in explaining variance in the outcome. In the example above, for each 0.270 unit drop in fat intake, LDL levels increase by 1 mg/dL unit, $P = 0.048$. For every 1.084 drop in the exercise scale, LDL increases by 1 mg/dL.

When visualizing a beta coefficient, think of a seesaw. Connie is on the right and Eddie is on the left. Connie is the outcome. Connie is in position 0, which is on the ground. Eddie is a potential predictor of a rise in Connie, from the ground to the highest point of 1. Eddie weighs less than Connie so when Eddie gets onto the seesaw, Connie only rises 0.75 or three-quarters the way off the ground, which means that Eddie's beta coefficient is 0.75. When we add Eddie's baby sister, Athena to his side, Connie rises up to a full 1, meaning that Athena's beta coefficient is 0.25.

Caveats

- Like the considerations for the logistic regression, not all statistically significant relationships that are found during the preliminary testing of your covariates (variables) should be considered for entry into your regression analysis; biologically, the relationship of the predictor may be meaningless in its relation to the outcome variable.
- A case record can only be included in your multivariable regression if it has valid values, i.e., no missing values, for the variables in the model (so choose wisely, so that you don't lose too many cases and thus lower your power to find an association).
- Selecting predictors to enter into a regression analysis: some, who don't know any better, may just enter all predictors into their regression analysis whether they make clinical sense or not and whether or not they are highly correlated with other predictors. This is not such a useful approach for many reasons.

Do not include predictors if:

- Your exploratory bivariate analyses of predictors and the outcome shows that the predictor had no association or correlation with LDL levels.
- The "predictor" has no biological association with the dependent outcome but may interact with another more important predictor that is also in the equation, thereby negating the strength of the more important predictor in predicting the outcome.
- The predictor is correlated highly with another predictor in the equation, so its co-presence may nullify the effect of both predictors in explaining the variance in LDL levels.

7.3.2   Multivariable vs. Multivariate Regression Analyses

Regression analyses can be performed in several ways, the most common of which are either multivariable or multivariate.

Multivariable regression:

$$Y = mX + b + \beta x_1 + \beta x_2 + \beta x_3 + \beta x_4 + \beta x_5.$$

Testing multiple predictors of an outcome.

Multivariate regression:

$$Y_1, Y_2, Y_3 = mX + b + \beta x_1.$$

Testing one set of predictors on multiple outcomes on the same patient or sample, as would be seen in a longitudinal study.

Again, this is one of those techniques where I would advise you to work with a statistician as the details go beyond the scope of this guide. Further reading on multivariable vs. multivariate analyses can be found online.[33]

Links to Online Tools

[31] https://people.emich.edu/aross15/coursepack3419/logistic-javascript.html

[32] https://sourceforge.net/projects/pspp4windows/files/2018-11-09/

[33] https://www.ncbi.nlm.nih.gov/pmc/articles/PMC3518362/

III Applied Statistics

8   Applied Statistics for the Laboratorian

It is often asked: "Which laboratory test is the best?" However, the best question to ask is, "Which test is best for my testing situation?" Obviously, there is no best test for all purposes; otherwise, all laboratories would exclusively use that one test. Of course, the utility of a test or how it is used in a testing strategy depends on the purpose of testing and the requirements within each specific testing situation, as well as the characteristics of the individual tests. Some tests perform better in certain geographic locations. For example, sera derived from one location may contain antibodies to a variety of parasitic organisms found in that area and, therefore, a particular test may produce a significant number of false-positive results. However, a different test that uses other antigens or a different test format may perform better in that particular geographic area (but not necessarily in other places). Also, the value of some tests may depend on the expertise of the laboratory workers and, therefore, a test must be chosen that can be performed accurately by those personnel.

All analytical methods are subject to different types of errors and variations. These create a certain degree of uncertainty in the results and, hence, affect the quality of results produced by the laboratory. Therefore, it is the responsibility of the laboratory to understand these variations and apply basic statistical and mathematical tools to define a test's performance characteristics and a test's limitations. Parameters are available that can be used to determine the relative usefulness or efficiency of a particular test, assuming that each test has been evaluated by properly trained individuals, performed exactly as required by the manufacturer, evaluated on the same sample of sera for which the test will ultimately be used, and performed under optimal testing conditions.

The test parameters that can assist in determining the usefulness of a test are sensitivity, specificity, efficiency, delta values, and predictive values. In addition, to further characterize a test's performance, it is important to assess its reproducibility and precision, and to determine whether the manufacturers produce tests that perform consistently (e.g., from lot to lot). Importantly, a valid evaluation must use a large enough sample size to minimize the chance of finding differences between the tests that are solely the result of random error (chance). The parameters used to describe a test's usefulness and accuracy are commonly known as "test indices," and each is discussed below.

In summary, although no one test may be best for all testing situations, the choice must reflect the needs of the population being tested, the infrastructure of the laboratory, the characteristics of the serum to be tested, and the performance of the test. This chapter describes the tools that can be used to evaluate test performance, but it must be emphasized that to define the performance characteristics of a test, all other parameters must be optimal and the testing conditions must meet the requirements of the test manufacturer.

8.1   Test Accuracy

Accuracy denotes the ability of an analytical method to obtain the "true" or "correct" result. The true result is sometimes referred to as the "target" result. Of course, attaining accuracy in a new method depends on knowing the true result. A major mistake that many investigators make when evaluating a new method is not having well-characterized samples; that is, not having samples that are known to be from infected or non-infected persons or, more correctly, containing the target marker or not. There must be no question as to the correct status of samples when determining the accuracy of a method. Test indices like sensitivity, specificity, positive and negative predictive value are all measures of test accuracy.

8.1.1   Sensitivity

The sensitivity of a diagnostic assay can refer to its analytical sensitivity or its epidemiologic sensitivity. The **analytical sensitivity** of a test is its ability to detect small quantities of the target, like HIV antibody, and tests with high analytical sensitivity are useful in samples where the incidence of HIV is high. Such tests may be expected to identify individuals who are in the earliest stages of infection. The **epidemiologic sensitivity** of a test describes its ability to correctly detect all samples containing the target analyte, i.e., infected persons in a sample who have established infection over a period of time where the target marker has fully evolved.

Because confirmatory assays may be less sensitive than screening tests, samples that are confirmed positive are most certainly from persons with established infection. A test's sensitivity can be calculated using the following formula:

$$\text{Sensitivity} = \frac{\text{True positives (infected persons detected by the test)}}{\text{All true positives (all infected persons)}} \times 100.$$

Another common and equivalent way of writing the formula is

$$\text{Sensitivity} = \frac{\text{True positives}}{\text{True positives} + \text{False negatives}} \times 100.$$

where true positives are the number of infected persons detected by the test, and false negatives are the number of infected persons who are incorrectly classified as negative by the test.

Sample:

1000	sera are tested
50	sera are from infected individuals
950	sera are from non-infected individuals

Test results: In comparison to the reference gold-standard testing (full characterization of the samples in a proven testing strategy), the test detects only 45 positives among the sera from the 50 individuals known to be HIV positive (i.e., the test produces five false-negative results). Therefore, the sensitivity is

$$\frac{45}{50} \times 100\%.$$

Thus, the sensitivity of the test is calculated to be 90%.

It is important to note that the method of characterizing the samples of "known" status is of utmost importance. What may be considered a standard or reference test, providing a correct result, may actually be less accurate than an investigational test under evaluation. Just because the test under evaluation yields a different result does not prove that it is wrong. Thus, when assessing sensitivity and specificity in evaluations, only samples whose status can be determined definitively should be used in the evaluation panel.

However, if a positive sample contains low levels of antibody, for example, and cannot be confirmed definitively, the status may be confirmed in subsequent bleeds from the subject as a verification that low levels of the analyte were present. The clinical status can be a guide, but the presence of the target analyte in the samples to be used in evaluations must be verified by serologic or molecular testing. Recall that a positive result alone by the test being evaluated (but negative by the reference test) can still represent a true positive if the test being evaluated is more sensitive than the reference test or tests being used to characterize the sample. Again, there must be no question as to the correct status of the samples that are used to determine test indices.

8.1.2   Specificity

The **specificity** of an assay is the ability of the test to correctly identify all individuals whose samples do not contain the target analyte (i.e., high-specificity assays produce no false-positive results). No screening assays for HIV are 100% specific and, therefore, the results must be confirmed using a more specific supplemental test or additional supplemental testing. The specificity of an assay can be calculated from the following formula:

$$\text{Specificity} = \frac{\text{True negatives}}{\text{All true negatives}} \times 100$$

where true negatives are non-infected persons classified as negative by the test and all true negatives are all non-infected persons.

Another way of writing the formula that is equivalent, is

$$\text{Specificity} = \frac{\text{True negatives}}{\text{True negatives} + \text{False positives}} \times 100$$

where true negatives are the number of non-infected persons classified as negative by the test, and false positives are the number of non-infected persons classified as positive by the test.

Sample:

1000 sera are tested

None are from infected persons.

In comparison to the reference test, the test under evaluation yields

5 sera give reactive results (i.e., five are false positives)

995 sera give negative results:

$$\frac{995}{1000} \times 100.$$

Thus, the specificity of the test is calculated to be 99.5%.

8.1.3   Test Efficiency

Test efficiency refers to the overall ability of a test to correctly identify all positive samples as positive and all negative samples as negative. That is, if a test is 100% efficient it will identify the status of all samples correctly with the absence of false-positive and false-negative results. As stated earlier, the test efficiency directly relates to test accuracy. Test efficiency reflects a combination of the sensitivity and the specificity of an assay and determines the total effectiveness of the assay in correctly identifying infected and non-infected persons (test accuracy). Test efficiency is determined as follows:

$$\text{Test efficiency} = \frac{\text{True positives} + \text{True negatives}}{\text{True positives} + \text{True negatives} + \text{False positives} + \text{False negatives}} \times 100.$$

Sample:

1000 sera tested

50 sera are from infected individuals

950 sera are from non-infected individuals.

Test results:

50 positive results (45 from the infected group and 5 false positive from the non-infected group)

950 negative results (945 from the non-infected group and 5 false negative from the infected group).

$$\frac{45+945}{45+945+5+5} \times 100\%.$$

Thus, the test efficiency is calculated to be 99%.

Although test efficacy can be a valuable assessment of how a test performs, in general, with true positives and true negatives, it can be misleading; for example, the test may produce no false-positive results, but a high number of false-negative results. In such cases, the efficacy may be fairly good, but the test is poor for determining true positives.

8.1.4   Predictive Values

Predictive values describe how a test of a given sensitivity and specificity might be expected to perform in one sample where the prevalence of infection in the sample being tested is known. Predictive values are principally epidemiological tools but may help in estimating how *frequently* a positive result is likely to represent a true result. Predictive values are estimated by knowing the test indices, sensitivity, and specificity, and the prevalence of the infection in a sample population. That is, they are dependent on the sensitivity and specificity of the test but also depend on the prevalence of the target antigen in the sample population, so that a ratio of expected correct results to all results is generated. The **positive predictive value (PPV)** is the ratio of positive results generated by the test (i.e., in infected persons) compared with the total number of positive results generated by the test (i.e., true positives plus false positives). Similar calculations are made for negative results in the sample. Therefore, the *value* of a test (i.e., the likelihood of a given result by the test being a correct result) may not depend on its sensitivity and specificity as much as it depends on the predictive values in the sample being tested. Therefore, the PPV is the likelihood that a positive result by the test is from an infected individual. The **negative predictive value (NPV)** is the likelihood that a negative result by the test is from a non-infected individual. Both PPV and NPV are influenced by prevalence and specificity or sensitivity, as will be illustrated below.

An example will illustrate the point. The predictive values are calculated as follows:

$$\text{Positive predictive value} = \frac{\text{True positives}}{\text{True positives} + \text{False positives}} \times 100\%;$$

$$\text{Negative predictive value} = \frac{\text{True negatives}}{\text{True negatives} + \text{False negatives}} \times 100\%.$$

The numerators, true positives and true negatives, are those that are detected by the test.

Sample #1 where the prevalence of infection is high (5%)

Sample:

2000 sera tested
100 sera are from infected individuals
1900 sera are from non-infected individuals.

A test is used that has a sensitivity of 99% and a specificity of 99%.

Test results:

118 positives could be expected (99 positives from the infected group with 1 false-negative result because of the 99% sensitivity, and 19 false positives from the non-infected group because of the 99% specificity).

1882 negatives could be expected (1881 negatives from the non-infected group because there were 19 false positives from this group and 1 false negative from the infected group).

Therefore, the predictive values are:

$$\text{PPV} = \frac{99}{99 + 19} \times 100\% = \frac{99}{118} \times 100\% = 83.9\%;$$

$$\text{NPV} = \frac{1881}{1881 + 1} \times 100\% = \frac{1881}{1882} \times 100\% = 99.9\%.$$

The chance of a positive result being from a truly infected person is 83.9%, and the chance of a negative result being from a truly non-infected person is 99.9%.

Now let's see how prevalence influences PPV and NPV, with the same percentage of false positives and false negatives (1%) in a different sample.

Sample #2 where the prevalence of infection is low (0.5%)

Sample:

2000 sera tested
10 sera are from infected individuals (prevalence of 0.5%)
1990 sera are from non-infected individuals.

The same test is used (sensitivity of 99% and specificity of 99%)

Test results:

10 positive results would be expected from the infected group (no false negatives with only 10 true positives [99% sensitivity of the test]).
19 false positives would be expected from the non-infected group (the specificity is 99%).

Therefore, there would be 29 positive results (10 from the infected group and 19 false positives from the non-infected group). There would be 1971 negative results by the test (all from the non-infected group, and no false negatives from the infected group).

Therefore, the predictive values are:

$$PPV = \frac{10}{10+19} \times 100\% = \frac{10}{29} \times 100\% = 34\%;$$

$$NPV = \frac{1971}{1971+0} \times 100\% = \frac{1971}{1971} \times 100\% = 100\%.$$

As shown, the same test (with the same specificity) yields the same number of false-positive results (19) but produces a different positive predictive value when testing these two samples from two populations with different prevalence rates. The chance of a positive result being from a truly infected individual is only 34% (10 true positives detected by the test and 19 false positives). This indicates that a positive result by the test will only be from an infected individual in about one out of three cases. Therefore, when a physician gets a reactive result from a single test from a laboratory, especially if derived from a sample that has a low prevalence, they should be cautious in what the result actually indicates if the concept of predictive values is not understood. In fact, it is more likely under these circumstances that the positive result is a *false* positive result! Therefore, the specificity of the test alone does not indicate the usefulness of the test, particularly in a low-prevalence population. The predictive value gives a more important understanding of what a positive or negative result actually means.

8.1.5   Coefficient of Variation

The **coefficient of variation** is another measure that describes dispersion of measurements in terms of the standard deviation from the mean. Functionally, it tests whether or not a test is precise and/or reproducible. It is commonly used in reproducibility and repeatability studies to determine how steady the measurements are (or are not) from an identical sample or person. Usually, if you are repeatedly testing the same sample over and over, it is preferred that the CV value is small. It is also commonly used to determine the repeatability of equipment; for example, a mechanical pipette delivers a finite volume (e.g., 20 μL), but does it deliver 20 μL every time? By measuring the volume delivered after multiple attempts, the variation (CV) can be determined. Most experts expect the CV of a pipette to be less than 10%.

The CV is calculated by dividing the SD by the mean of a distribution which is derived from the same sample or subject:

$$\text{CV for a sample} = \text{SD}/\bar{x},$$

where SD is the standard deviation and $\bar{x}$ is the sample mean.

Using the equation above, the mean (5.25) and SD (5.06) gives a CV of 0.96, or 96%, which is quite high. Keep in mind that this calculation of CV is only appropriate for normally distributed measurement data, meaning that one would not normally calculate a mean or standard deviation or a CV for heavily skewed data (Section 1.5.6).

Example for the Laboratorian

Keith and Lori have each been given 10 replicate aliquots of blood from *one healthy volunteer* to test for cholesterol. Both technicians performed their tests using the same measurement procedure, the same measuring instrument under the same conditions, in the same location, and the test repetition occurred over a short period of time.

Keith gets a mean of 92 and a standard deviation of 2.5.
Lori gets a mean of 94 and a standard deviation of 2.3.

Which technician had better test repeatability?

$$\text{Keith CV} = \frac{2.5}{92} \times 100\% = 2.7\%.$$

$$\text{Lori CV} = \frac{2.3}{94} \times 100\% = 2.4\%.$$

So, Lori was able to produce more consistent results as demonstrated by having a lower CV than Keith's, meaning that Lori demonstrated better test repeatability. This could be because Lori had better pipetting technique. However, repeat analysis by one technician (with constant technique) will most likely reflect the inherent reproducibility or precision of the pipette itself.

8.2   Sample Size for Determining Test Indices

8.2.1   Establishing Sensitivity and Specificity: Taking Prevalence into Account

I am developing a non-invasive HIV test for which I would like to determine the sensitivity and specificity. The rapid, saliva-based test can be used in public testing venues such as churches, community centers, and health fairs, and results can be obtained in as little as 10–15 minutes. If the patients test positive, I will refer them to a clinic where they can seek treatment and care.

An important note about how the Food and Drug Administration (FDA) will accept or reject an assay for approval: they set up strict guidelines that the experimental test must adhere to, to be considered for their seal of approval. Rather than being concerned about where to set power, alpha, and beta, they are more concerned about test accuracy, which, in a sense, is power. They may ask that the test perform as well as or better than the currently used gold-standard assay, which happens to have 99% sensitivity and specificity, and an error margin of just 2%, meaning that the FDA will allow a misclassification in just 2% of the samples tested, setting the lower bound of the confidence interval at 98%.

How do I proceed?

First, a gold-standard test (reference test) must be chosen for comparison with the test being investigated (experimental test). In the USA, an FDA-approved test is usually the reference test because it has been thoroughly and appropriately evaluated. For our example, let's choose a reference test that has been validated to have a sensitivity of 99%. Note that the discussion below will refer to evaluating the sensitivity of an experimental test; the exact same calculations would be applied for evaluating the specificity of a test.

Our goal is to determine if the experimental test has the same sensitivity as the reference test, i.e., if the performance of the experimental test is within the confidence intervals of the reference test. So, we shall think of this as being a test of equivalence or of non-inferiority, and we will set the lower bound of our 95% confidence interval to at least 0.98 (98%). In other words, after the evaluation is complete and the confidence interval established, the experimental test must have a sensitivity at a level where the CI range will not be less than 98%. If this is the case, then it can be expected (within statistical confidence) that the experimental test will have an "equivalent" sensitivity to the reference test.

In addition to those parameters, we must introduce another parameter – the "power" that the calculation and conclusion will yield. Power can be thought of as the degree of certainty of our evaluation (that the tests have equivalent sensitivity) and this can be set at a percent. For example, most authorities set the power of an evaluation such as this at 80%. However, choosing a power of 90% would give more certainty about the conclusions, but would require a larger sample size.

Thus, to determine the sensitivity of the experimental test, we need to select a number of positive samples to test using both the reference test and the experimental test. Importantly, the sample size to select will depend on whether you have archived positive samples to use (known positives), or whether you will be testing a population of persons with unknown status (the number of persons who are positive is not known). In the latter case, the number of persons to test to arrive at an adequate sample size of positives will depend on the prevalence of positives in the population. In most situations, the true prevalence will not be known; however, it can usually be estimated. In the discussion below, we will show the sample size calculations (1) for evaluating the test when using known positive samples, and (2) when we want to evaluate the test in the field with a population where the prevalence is not known but estimated. You will see that the sample sizes needed are dramatically different.

(1) **For evaluating a test with known positive samples:**
   - Let's use a tool to calculate power and sample size.[34]
   - Let's set the confidence interval at 0.95 (or 95%).
   - The expected proportion is 0.99, which is the reported sensitivity of the reference test.
   - The width of the confidence interval we will set is 0.02; this means that I am setting the 95% confidence interval to be 0.98–1.0. Again, the lower bound of the 95% confidence interval cannot be lower than 0.98 (or 98%) for the two tests to be considered equivalent; that is, the tests will not be considered equivalent if the lower bound is less than 98%. In most FDA clinical trials, the FDA wants to see this level of performance and certainly for a test to be approved.
   - Then, press "Calculate."

Note that when sensitivity or specificity is approaching 0 or 1, such as 0.99, we want to use the binomial "exact" calculator result as the result of choice. If the sensitivity moves towards 0.5, use the results from the normal approximation to the binomial calculation.

Result: The number of HIV-positive samples on which we need to conduct our non-inferiority study for the saliva test is 499 samples. At 99% sensitivity, we expect that 494 of those samples will test positive.

(2) **For evaluating a test with a population where the prevalence is not known but estimated:**

But wait, we are screening! Not everyone is positive, so we must test it in the field!

Now, we need to know the prevalence of disease (see Figure 8.1). If we surmise that the prevalence is around 1%, then to get 494 positive samples, we would need to screen 497/0.01 (= 49,700) HIV-positive and HIV-negative people, again, if this is indeed a field study.

Now, let's see what happens when sensitivity, specificity, confidence intervals, and precision (width of CI) vary.

Let's calculate the sample size after we retain the 95% CI, increase the sensitivity of the test to 99.5%, reduce the total width of the confidence interval to 1%, and retain a prevalence of 1%:

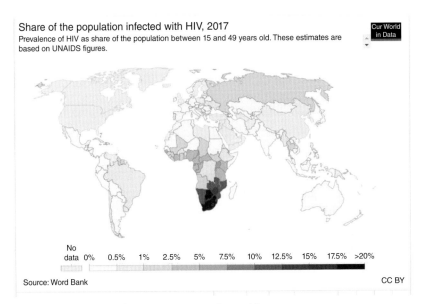

Share of the population infected with HIV, 2017
Prevalence of HIV as share of the population between 15 and 49 years old. These estimates are based on UNAIDS figures.

No data 0%   0.5%   1%   2.5%   5%   7.5%   10%   12.5%   15%   17.5%   >20%

Source: Word Bank   CC BY

Figure 8.1 Prevalence of HIV/AIDS across the world.

Confidence interval = 95% CI
Anticipated sensitivity = 99.5% = 0.995
Anticipated specificity = 99.5% = 0.995
CI width = 0.01 (you are setting the 95% CI to 0.995–1.005)
Estimated prevalence = 1%.

We enter everything into the equation to calculate sample size.

We will need to screen 1001 persons; at the 99.5% level of sensitivity, this will give us 10 HIV-positive specimens.

Now that the HIV prevalence in this area is 1%, the number of HIV-positive and HIV-negative persons that you must screen in the field is 996/0.01 = 99,600.

So, increasing the sensitivity has made a significant increase in sample size!

But now, let's tighten the confidence interval from 95% to 99%:

Confidence interval = 99% CI
Anticipated sensitivity = 99.5% = 0.995
Anticipated specificity = 99.5% = 0.995
CI width = 0.01 (you are setting the 95% CI to 0.995–1.005)
Estimated prevalence = 1%.

The tightening of the confidence interval has resulted in the increase of sample size from 1001 to 1595 HIV-positive persons, which at 99.5% sensitivity will correctly identify 1 HIV-positive sample; accordingly, 1587/0.01 or 158,700 HIV-positive and HIV-negative persons will need to be screened when the prevalence is 1%.

Okay, now let's see what happens when we loosen the width of the confidence interval from 0.01 to 0.02:

Confidence interval = 95% CI
Anticipated sensitivity = 99% = 0.99
Anticipated specificity = 99% = 0.99
CI width = 0.02 (you are setting the 95% CI to 0.98–1.00)
Estimated prevalence = 1%.

So, compared to the very first example above, loosening the width of the confidence interval resulted in screening 230 persons; at the 99.5% level of sensitivity, this will give us 2 HIV-positive specimens.

Now that the HIV prevalence in this area is 1%, the number of HIV-positive and HIV-negative persons that you must screen in the field is 228/0.01 = 22,800.

So, loosening the width of the confidence interval decreased the number of necessary persons on which to test your assay.

Now, let's take the same example as above, and increase the prevalence rate of HIV and see how that impacts the number of HIV-positive and HIV-negative persons we must screen:

Confidence interval = 95% CI
Anticipated sensitivity = 99% = 0.99
Anticipated specificity = 99% = 0.99
CI width = 0.05 (you are setting the 95% CI to 0.995–1.00)
Estimated prevalence = 5%.

But now we want to screen 228/0.05 or 4560 persons.

Increasing prevalence of the disease will lower the necessary sample size when tested in the field of positives and negatives (see Table 8.1).

So, it is also important to know the prevalence of the disease to be screened for before setting up your screening study.

Unfortunately, there is no online tool that calculates sample size for this situation, so you may want to speak with a statistician about this, or if you so dare, do it yourself!

Table 8.1 Example of sample sizes for varying prevalence and confidence intervals

Prevalence	Sensitivity/specificity	Power	Precision	CI	No. required
0.01	0.995 sensitivity	0.90	0.01	0.95	1,890
0.01	0.995 specificity	0.90	0.01	0.95	19
0.01	0.995 sensitivity	0.90	0.01	0.99	33,100
0.01	0.995 specificity	0.90	0.01	0.99	348
0.05	0.995 sensitivity	0.90	0.01	0.95	3,780
0.05	0.995 specificity	0.90	0.01	0.95	200
0.05	0.995 sensitivity	0.90	0.01	0.99	6,220
0.05	0.995 specificity	0.90	0.01	0.99	348
0.20	0.995 sensitivity	0.90	0.01	0.95	945
0.20	0.995 specificity	0.90	0.01	0.95	237
0.20	0.995 sensitivity	0.90	0.01	0.99	3,310
0.20	0.995 specificity	0.90	0.01	0.99	414

8.2.2 Establishing Sensitivity and Specificity: Without Taking Prevalence into Account

Now, rather than calculating sample size in field studies with differing prevalence rates, let's move to situations where you must test known positive and known negative specimens, so it is not a field study where prevalence is of concern.

When calculating sample size for comparing two proportions, it is simply that prevalence is not involved because, like the example of comparing two proportions, it is simply a matter of entering the proportions into the online calculator.[35]

So, you can see how this sample size and power machine operates:

- Increase precision → increase sample size.
- Tighten confidence intervals → increase sample size.
- Increase power → increase sample size.
- Increase sample size → increase power.

And the reverse of all these interactions will follow suit.

8.3   Test Validation

Test validation is a term used to describe a series of methodically performed procedures to measure the accuracy and precision of a test; validation studies are usually done in comparison to a test that is already licensed and in use. A valid test is that which is found to perform within clinically acceptable limits. There are a number of ways to measure the accuracy of a test, namely by assessing its validity, reliability, test–retest reliability, precision studies, reproducibility studies, inter- and intra-lot variation.

No assay will produce exactly the same quantitative results when repeated multiple times, because (1) many variables can change slightly during the same run, e.g., pipetting, instrument variability, antigen coating in different wells or cartridges, inconsistent washes between wells, and (2) random error occurs. This is one reason why confidence limits are incorporated into parameters when determining the performance characteristics of a test. Random errors are inconsistencies that occur for unknown or unidentified reasons. For example, a pipette might perform inconsistently between samples, or one pipette tip might be malformed, resulting in a random error. Random errors may be reflected in the precision assessment of an assay and will be inconsistent, whereas systematic errors (e.g., if a pipette were not properly calibrated) will be noted by consistently abnormal results (either higher or lower than expected).

8.3.1   Validity vs. Reliability

Validity is a term that is used to describe the ability of a test to accurately detect the agent it is intended to detect. If a test is developed to detect *E. coli* in samples, but it only detects known positive samples 30% of the time, we would say that the validity of the *E. coli* test is poor. **Reliability**, in contrast, refers to the degree to which a detection test is consistent and stable in what the test is designed to measure. The reliability of a diagnostic test is critical to its quality and utility. If test components (e.g., reagents) are stored at higher temperatures than recommended, it is likely that the test will become unreliable and will be of little value. If the test is performed on the same sample that produces consistent results on 100% of the runs, it is known to be highly reliable, but that's only if the test also has good validity. However, systematic errors can produce results that are consistently incorrect, which would reduce the validity but with no effect on its corresponding reliability.

8.3.2   Test–Retest Reliability

Test–retest reliability is the most common type of reliability measure that is applied in laboratory settings. It represents the stability and consistency of test performance. For example, if we were to test cholesterol levels in the same individuals on two occasions, preferably at the same hour, by the same technician in the same environment to remove any bias, we would hope that the measurements would be similar. But how do we know that the test results are or are not identical?

Mathematically, the formula for measuring the test–retest reliability is $(C - D)/(C + D)$, where C = concordant pairs and D = discordant pairs. So, let's say we are measuring the test–retest reliability of an assay that gives binary results (positive/negative):

Run 1	Run 2	Concordant (C)	Discordant (D)
0	0		
1	1		
0	1	3	2
0	0		
1	0		

$$\text{Test}-\text{retest reliability} = \frac{C - D}{C + D} = \frac{3 - 2}{3 + 2} = \frac{1}{5} = 0.20,$$

which is a pretty weak correlation.

Would you consider that test to be reliable when its test–retest reliability is 0.2? Of course not! But we only compared five values. Running a proper sample size calculation to hypothesize that the test has 80% power to detect a test–retest reliability value of, say, 0.96 will give you the number of samples you should test to find the test's true reliability. You can enter these numbers into the WebPower sample size calculator[36] (Figure 8.2).

8.3.3   Precision (Intra-run Variability) and Reproducibility (Inter-run Variability)

Precision usually refers to the ability of a test to produce the same result when a sample is tested multiple times simultaneously (i.e., on the same run); this is also referred to as the *intra-run variability* (within the same run) of the test. Precision refers to "short-term" repeatability at the

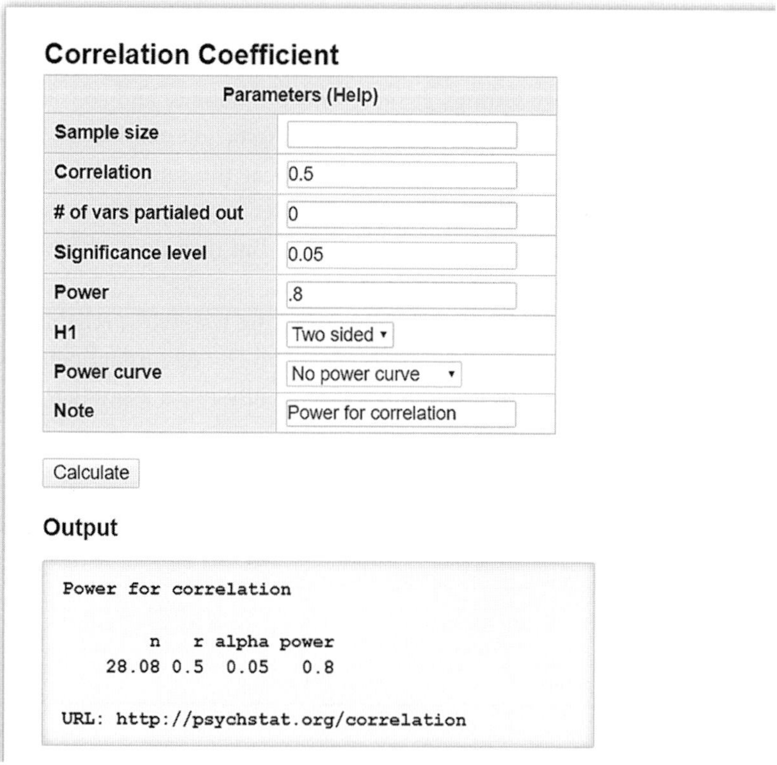

Correlation Coefficient

Parameters (Help)	
Sample size	
Correlation	0.5
# of vars partialed out	0
Significance level	0.05
Power	.8
H1	Two sided ▾
Power curve	No power curve ▾
Note	Power for correlation

Calculate

Output

```
Power for correlation

       n    r alpha power
   28.08 0.5  0.05   0.8

URL: http://psychstat.org/correlation
```

Figure 8.2 Free online sample size calculator.

same location under very similar conditions, whether testing is within the same run or between different runs.

Precision can be expressed as the fraction of concordant results over all results (for tests producing a binary outcome) and as a mean and standard deviation (for tests producing a quantitative result). If the test produces results on a log scale, be sure to normalize your data before calculating the mean and SD.

Testing replicating the same samples on the same test run, at the same location, will assess the precision of a test. It is recommended that at least 10 replicates be included from each of 10 different samples (including several positive samples and, preferably, using one weakly positive sample). If a quantitative test, such as an ELISA, is used, a mean and standard deviation of the OD readings can be calculated from the resultant OD reading to have some idea of variability. If a rapid test is used, the reactions can be scored from 0 to 4+ for each replicate and non-parametric analyses may be used to assess the results. For samples around the cutoff (low levels of antibodies), it could be expected that the results may show considerable variability. For example, if a sample is on the border of reactive/non-reactive, the testing of replicates (even if tested 200 times) might be expected to produce results below the cutoff half of the time. If using samples with low, but not too low, levels of antibodies, a test should yield the same outcome in terms of status. If the precision of multiple tests is to be compared, samples where the variability can be gauged should be used.

Reproducibility can be considered as the ability to achieve the same results with the same test, on different days at the same location, or on different days at different locations (with different equipment and technologists):

$$\text{Reproducibility} = \frac{\text{No. test results differing between days}}{\text{Total no. tests performed on same no. samples on 20 days}} \times 100\%.$$

The lower the calculated number, the better is the reproducibility of a particular test. Statistical tools can be used to determine if the differences are "statistically significant." It is important when performing reproducibility studies to be sure that the samples are appropriately prepared. Specifically, frozen aliquots of the same sample must be maintained, and one thawed and tested each day. This is to minimize any effects on the assay that might be produced with extra freeze–thaw cycles or by one sample remaining in the refrigerator for many days. Figure 8.3 illustrates the differences between precision, reproducibility, and accuracy.

The arrows indicate repeated attempts to hit the middle of the target (the true value). The target center is the "true value." If the result is the true value, the result is accurate. If several replicates of a sample deliver the true result, it is accurate and precise. If the result from the same sample after a number of runs at a different location delivers the same result, it is reproducible, whether accurate or not. Alternatively, a measurement can be quite precise or reproducible, but it can be very inaccurate!

8.3.4   Inter-lot Variation

Test kits are usually sent in units called lots, which may contain anywhere from 25 to 100 kits. It is important to know the performance characteristics of your test kits before using them in the field. One measure that expresses these characteristics is **inter-lot variation**. This can be assessed by running

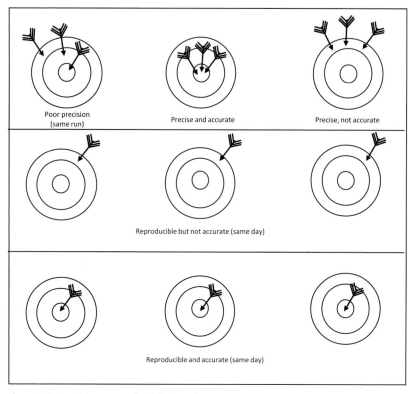

Figure 8.3 Precision, reproducibility, and accuracy.

the same samples, by the same technician, under the same conditions to see if the results are the same. If they are not the same, the variation is likely due to the lots; of course, one must first determine that each lot shows good precision and reproducibility. That is, if the pipette is not precise, the variability in the lot might be the inconsistency of the pipette!

8.3.5   Intra-lot Variation

When receiving test kits in bulk, it is always wise to measure the variation of results after running tests multiple times on the same kit lot. We do this to measure **intra-lot**, or within-lot, variation. After ruling out technician error and random error, you might return the kits to the manufacturer if you find an unacceptable error rate of >1%, for example.

Again, whether the test results are quantitative or binary, summarizing the inter- or intra-lot variation can be expressed as the mean and standard deviation, or the number of concordant results/all results, respectively.

8.4   Interpreting Pharmacokinetics and Pharmacodynamics Data

Pharmacokinetics is the study of drug absorption, distribution, metabolism, and excretion and the time it takes to reach these processes. A pharmacokinetics plot illustrates the concentration of drug in plasma on the y-axis (C_P) and time on the x-axis, as shown in Figure 8.4. The area under the curve (AUC) is a measure of the total area between the curve and the x- and y-axes; ranging from zero to infinity, the AUC is a measure of total drug exposure through the kinetic processes.

Pharmacodynamics, in contrast, describes the relationship between drug concentration and the concentration of drug-specific receptors. Let's take the example in Figure 8.5. This pharmaceutical company's goal is to develop a drug that is effective for a disease but at the same time, it minimizes spikes in blood pressure. The chart shows the effect of adding an adjuvant Drug X to norepinephrine and showing the biologic response in blood pressure.

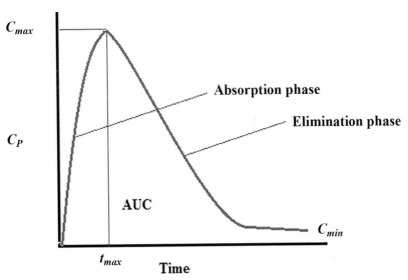

Figure 8.4 Graphic of the pharmacokinetic process.

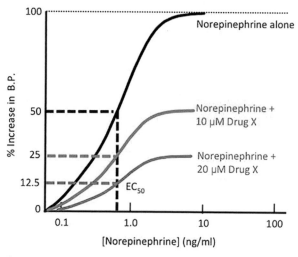

Figure 8.5 Graphic of the pharmacodynamic process.

Links to Online Tools

[34] http://www.sample-size.net/sample-size-conf-interval-proportion/

[35] https://webpower.psychstat.org/models/prop02/.

[36] https://webpower.psychstat.org/models/cor01/

9 Applied Statistics for the Clinician

As most concepts and statistical tools have already been described in previous chapters, the tools described in this chapter are specific to the clinician and epidemiologist working in the field to describe disease burden and population characteristics. It is also important for clinicians to understand these concepts as they review peer-reviewed medical journal articles, so that they don't simply skip over the statistical methods section.

9.1 Prevalence of Disease

Prevalence is the number of persons with a disease (old cases and new cases) divided by the number of individuals in the population during a specified time period. So, if we are speaking of the prevalence of coronavirus in Baltimore City schools, the number of actual coronavirus cases in the schools would be the numerator and the total number of school attendees and staff at the schools in Baltimore City would represent the denominator; note that all pupils and staff are at risk of being exposed to the virus.

Prevalence represents a slice of the population in terms of, for example, disease prevalence at one time point (point prevalence) or during one period (period prevalence). Of course, the number of persons at risk of disease varies across regions/states and other comparison strata, so when we are making comparisons across regions, for example, we usually express prevalence rates of rare diseases in units of N per 1,000,000 population. When we are not comparing rates between demographic or geographic strata, we might simply state the number of disease cases divided by the total number at risk in that one region or stratum:

$$\frac{\text{Total number of existing cases}}{\text{Total number in the population}} \times 100.$$

However, there are circumstances when the denominator is not necessarily the number at risk for the disease. When we express the prevalence of an autosomal dominant genetic disease like Huntington's Disease, for example, the only persons at risk are those who have a parent with Huntington's Disease, but that would be a difficult number to obtain. Thus, it is understood that we express prevalence rates of Huntington's Disease and any other genetic disease in rates per 1,000,000 at-risk and not-at-risk persons, as most genetic diseases are fairly rare (by the way, the prevalence of Huntington's Disease in the USA is somewhere between the 95% CI of 4.1 to 5.2 per 100,000).

Point prevalence is the rate of cases at one given time point, whereas **period prevalence** is the rate of cases (new and existing) during a specified time period.

You may also see age-adjusted prevalence and incidence rates, which stratify the values by age. Let's take an example that might be obvious.

Age-Adjusted Prevalence Rates of Alzheimer's Disease

The CDC publishes the *Morbidity and Mortality Weekly Report* (MMWR) in which they track rates of death from Alzheimer's Disease from 1990–2014. As shown in Figure 9.1 and Table 9.1, the numbers per 1,000,000 population are increasing substantially, especially for those greater than or equal to age 85, which is to be expected.

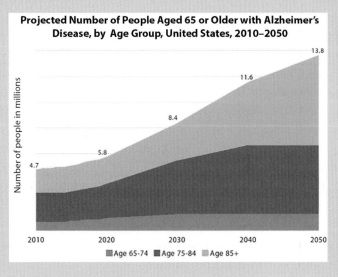

Figure 9.1 Age-stratified prevalence.

Table 9.1 Age-adjusted prevalence

Age group	No. in group	No. with Alzheimer's Disease	Age-stratified prevalence
≤64	100,000	2	2/100,000
65–74	100,000	4	4/100,000
75–84	100,000	174	174/100,000
≥85	100,000	996	996/100,000

9.2   Incidence of Disease

Incidence, in contrast, is the number of new cases of disease or newly diagnosed cases of disease within a defined time period. Estimated over time, it is the prevalence of disease divided by time. It can be expressed in percentages as the number of new infections during a specified time period, divided by the total population at risk at the start of the time interval. Standardized, it can be expressed in terms of cases per 1000 or 1,000,000 population.

But again, is that "population at risk"? If, for example, you do not participate in risky behavior, you are probably not at risk for HIV or HCV. However, we must exclude some cases from the numerator if indeed an infant was perinatally infected through his mother or an individual contracted HIV or HCV through a blood transfusion, since they are not part of the denominator, that is, they were not at risk. One would simply need to specify the denominator when stating such a rate and specify the time period during which the number of new cases was measured. For these reasons, genetic diseases are usually expressed in terms of prevalence, whereas rates of infectious diseases are often expressed in terms of incidence.

One may see the incidence of a certain condition increasing because more diagnostic testing is occurring in the field, results are generated more rapidly, and newer tests are better able to detect an analyte or better discriminate disease from non-disease. For these reasons, true incidence can be a tricky parameter to estimate. Sometimes, the incidence of an infectious disease can be difficult to estimate as many infected individuals will not know that they are infected until they begin to develop noticeable symptoms. Simply surveilling a population to measure the number of new cases of HIV will inevitably miss the majority of cases that have not consulted with a physician for testing since they have not yet developed the tell-tale symptoms (night sweats, fever, lethargy, sore throat, to name a few). For this reason, we must rely on diagnostic tests that detect markers of the disease, such as their immune response (the appearance of the HIV antibody response to the HIV antigen). The same is true for malaria and Lyme Disease, where symptoms may not appear for weeks or months while the virus/bacterium is incubating. For these reasons, disease incidence can be difficult to estimate, but physicians and other scientists should know the disease epidemiology before attempting to make such estimates. Like prevalence, incidence can also be stratified by age or any other logical demographic strata, such as income quartile or race.

Incidence density is mathematically different from incidence rate. In the denominator, incidence density incorporates how much time each person has contributed to the cohort.

Let's take, for example, the incidence density of HCV in a population of methadone clinic attendees over a 1-year period; that is, the rate of new cases of disease among clinic attendees over a 1-year period.

The number of new cases in 1 year is still the numerator, but the denominator is different. The denominator is expressed as how long each person was in the methadone cohort, which is better known as a calculation of "person-time.":

Client	How long in clinic	HCV+ or −
A	9/12 months	+
B	6/12 months	−
C	2/12 months	−
D	6/12 months	+
E	9/12 months	+
F	2/12 months	−

Sum: 34 person-months (which becomes the denominator of the incidence density equation).

- We know that three became HCV-positive during their stay.
- So, the incidence density, or the incidence rate of new HCV infections in the methadone clinic, is 3/34 = 0.088.
- Or 8.8% per 34 person-months (which is the person-time measurement).

Now, if we had incorrectly calculated incidence by the number who became HCV-positive by the total number of clients, that would have come to 3/6, or 500/1000, which we know is vastly wrong.

9.3   Morbidity Rate

Morbidity rate (as opposed to mortality rate) refers to the rate of disease or disability in a population or by population strata. Disease is highlighted as many think of "morbid" as being deceased, when indeed the Latin term *morbosus* means diseased, sickly, unhealthy, etc. Morbidity can be caused by any number of chronic or acute conditions, or caused by certain treatments. Likened to prevalence and incidence rates, morbidity is expressed as a ratio of diseased to the total number at risk of the disease. Well, doesn't that sound like the definition of prevalence? You're right! It is!

$$\frac{\text{Number with the disease}}{\text{Number at risk of getting the disease}} \times 100.$$

Diabetes Morbidity Rate in the USA

What was the diabetes morbidity rate in the USA in 2018? The denominator would be equal to all US residents, since we are all eventually at risk of this chronic condition. The US Census Bureau[37] reports that the population estimate in 2018 was 327,167,434. In 2018, the number of persons diagnosed with diabetes was 13,567,000 females and 13,710,000 males (total = 27,277,000), as reported by the United Health Foundation.[38] So, dividing the numerator by the denominator gives 27,277,000/327,167,434 × 100 = 8.3%.

Morbidity rates can also be stratified by any demographic or clinical feature such as race, gender, age group, or body mass index groupings.

9.4   Mortality Rate

Mortality rate, in contrast, refers to the number of deaths divided by the number at risk of death, which would be everyone unless a demographic stratum was specified, or if one is not at risk, as in genetically acquired diseases.

$$\frac{\text{Number of deaths}}{\text{Number at risk of death}} \times 100.$$

Well, really, we are all at risk of death no matter how young we are, so the denominator of a mortality rate is usually the size of the population. However, when measuring mortality rate for ovarian cancer, the number at risk of death includes women only. So, again, be careful when choosing your denominators as they can be tricky to select correctly.

Diabetes Mortality Rate in the USA

The number of deaths from diabetes in the USA in 2018 was approximately 70,341. Divided by the number of persons living in the US in 2018 (327,167,434), we get (70,341/327,167,434) × 100 = 0.0215%.

9.5   Quality Improvement vs. Research Studies

Quality improvement (QI) studies can sometimes be difficult to distinguish from research studies. Why is it important to make this distinction? Because QI projects normally do not require IRB approval, while most research projects do. According to America's Federal Code of Regulations, research is defined as "a systematic investigation, including research development, testing and evaluation, designed to develop or contribute to generalizable knowledge" that can be transferred to other populations or settings, while QI projects are intended to quantify improvements to patients' care and processes of care using pre- vs. post-interventional data. Well, how does any of this relate to statistics?

Research usually produces patient-level data, while QI studies normally produce aggregated data that must be analyzed differently. Without getting into the intricacies of how QI data are analyzed and applied to healthcare settings, the statistical analysis of research data usually results in a research publication. Thus, it is paramount that one understands the statistical methods used to complete the project and how to state the results appropriately.

9.6   Clinical Trials – Intention to Treat

When designing the statistical methods of clinical trials, it is important to understand the concept of the term "intention to treat." **Intention to treat** is a method whereby one includes all enrolled participants in the analysis dataset, regardless of whether the participant was ever randomized to experimental drug or placebo, whether or not they were non-compliant, and whether or not they dropped out before the trial was completed. There are a few pros and cons, however, in applying this concept. Assuming dropouts may occur at similar rates in the experimental group and in the placebo group, the application of the intention to treat concept should not bias the outcome measures in one direction or the other, and it provides a full accounting of all outcomes for all enrollees. The downside of this concept is that enrollees who never complied with taking their assigned treatment tend to dilute the effect of the outcome measurement. However, it is worthwhile discussing this concept with your study team at the clinical trial design stage.

9.7   Correcting Sample Size for Losses to Follow-Up

On the same note, when designing your sample size, it is also important to consider rates of losses to follow-up during the duration of the clinical trials, or any research endeavor. The length of the study may also dictate how many losses to expect per month or per year, which will drive up the need to enroll more patients. Of course, this can also occur in a laboratory setting where some samples may be lost, non-viable, or of insufficient quantity or quality. Thus, after calculating sample size, it is wise to add, say, 5% more patients or samples to correct for losses to follow-up.

9.8   Public Use Files

Another treasure trove of data is available for free or at cost from a number of medical networks. These very large, patient-level datasets are de-identified and are careful to remove all protected health information, and are thus deemed to be exempt from IRB review. These databases are designed to provide for valuable quality improvement data analyses.

A few of these network databases are described below.

Healthcare Cost and Utilization Project (HCUP) databases

- The National Inpatient Sample (NIS) database represents a 20% sampling of all hospital discharges across the USA, totaling about 7 to 8 million discharges per year.

- The State Inpatient Database (SID) represents admissions and 30-day readmissions within US states participating in HCUP.

National Surgical Quality Improvement Program (NSQIP)

- The NSQIP data provides a wealth of research opportunities. These data pertain to surgical procedures and contain more granular detail than NIS. Available surgical quality-improvement databases are:

Cardiac	Orthopedics
General	Otolaryngology
Gynecological	Plastics
Interventional Radiology	Thoracic
Neurosurgery	Vascular
Urology	

Metabolic and Bariatric Surgical Accreditation and Quality Improvement Program (MBSAQIP)

- The American College of Surgeons (ACS) and the American Society for Metabolic and Bariatric Surgery (ASMBS) combined their respective national bariatric surgery accreditation programs into a single unified program to achieve one national accreditation standard for bariatric surgery centers, the MBSAQIP, which is available for our use.

National Cancer Databases (NCDBs)

- Additionally, the ACS have coordinated efforts to provide cancer-specific NCDBs which offer a wealth of cancer registry data that may be used to answer important research questions.

Links to Online Tools

[37] https://www.census.gov/quickfacts/fact/table/US/PST120218
[38] https://www.americashealthrankings.org/explore/annual/measure/Diabetes/state/ALL

10   Interpreting Graphs and Charts

A few general notes about graphs and charts. In every diagram, please
include:

- legends
- axis labels
- axis measurements
- units of measurement
- titles
- footnotes.

There are many graphs and charts displayed on the TV news that don't carry
legends or units of measurement, rendering the chart absolutely useless! Even
if you can fully interpret your graph or chart, wonder if others will be able to
make the same interpretations. Some graphs and charts can be somewhat
intimidating, so it is best to have consistently clear labels and legends.

10.1   Normal Curve

One thing that can truly stump any student is the instructor's assumption
that the student knows what the **normal curve** is or what it means. Stated
as simply as possible, the x-axis is the value of the variable and the y-axis is
the probability that the x-values will occur in your sample or in the
universe of values. You can see that the normal distribution in
Figure 10.1 centers perfectly around 0 (which is the mean) and within
two standard deviations (2SD) of the mean. Technically, the y-axis is the
normal probability density function (PDF). When plotting a **histogram** of
your data, you will easily see if your data adhere to a normal distribution or
tilt to the left or right, or are log-distributed. It is at this point that you

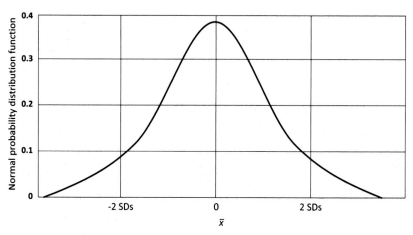

Figure 10.1 Normal probability plot.

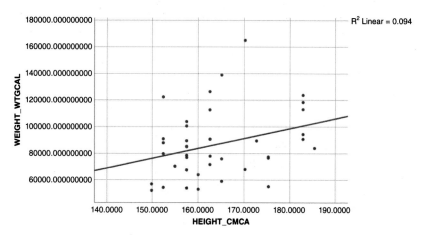

Figure 10.2 Scatterplot.

decide to either transform your data to meet a normal distribution or to use non-parametric statistics on your data.

10.2   Scatterplots

Scatterplots provide useful information regarding the relationship between two variables, one variable on the *y*-axis and the other on the *x*-axis. As you can see in Figure 10.2, the relationship between height and

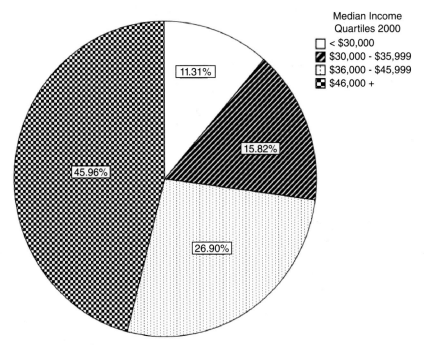

Figure 10.3 Pie chart.

weight is linear with a few outliers. As scatterplots cannot give quantitative measures such as correlation coefficients (Section 4.3.3) and regression coefficients (Section 7.3.1), they may be used as pictorial representations of bivariate relationships.

10.3   Pie Charts

Very simply, **pie charts** (Figure 10.3) illustrate univariate characteristics of a single ordinal (Section 6.2) or nominal (Section 6.3) variable. Pie charts give useful, visual glances at data distributions.

10.4   Bar Graphs

Bar graphs can illustrate nominal (including binary) or ordinal data on the x-axis and count or percentage data on the y-axis. As shown in Figure 10.4, we are looking at the number or percentage of individuals in racial groups (y-axis)

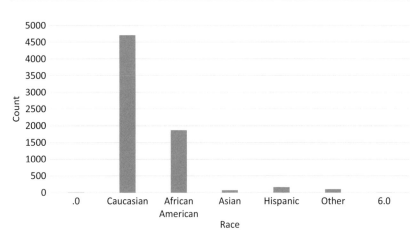

Figure 10.4 Bar graph.

as represented by bars, while the *x*-axis shows the race category. Note that the difference between the bar chart and the **histogram** is that the *x*-axis for the bar chart contains nominal or ordinal categories while the *x*-axis of the histogram contains continuous data. Thus, the histogram is appropriate for determining distributional normality of a continuous variable, but the bar chart is not.

10.5   Boxplots

Alternatively, **boxplots** are another pictorial representation of how data are distributed between groups. The boxplot also gives a wealth of information. In the boxplot in Figure 10.5, the *x*-axis shows two values for one variable (sex), and the *y*-axis gives values of another variable (weight). In this case, we are looking at weights in a bariatric population for males and females, and it is clear from these depictions that males are significantly heavier than females. Here we also show the interquartile ranges, the 95% confidence intervals, the means, and the outliers (small circles above the 95% upper bound). That's a lot of information to pack into a simple diagram! This type of graph can be used on any set of data containing continuous data (e.g., weight) and nominal or ordinal data (e.g., gender or Likert scale data, respectively). When you have multiple groups on the *x*-axis, you can draw lines between the groups to show the *P*-value resulting from the comparison of the means, as shown in Figure 10.5.

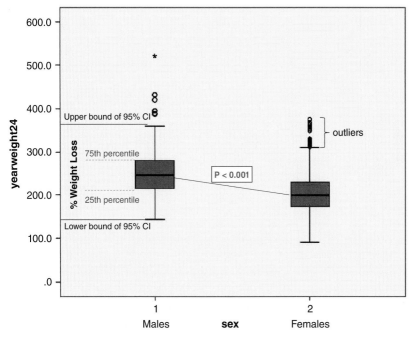

Figure 10.5 Boxplot.

10.6   Line Graphs

Line graphs can also serve as great portrayals of relationships of one, or between two or more groups (Figure 10.6). It is clearly seen that although both males and females stay in hospital an average of 24 hours after surgery, there are many more males than females that stay for 24 hours.

10.7   Forest Plots

You might recall back in Section 6.1.2, when we were discussing odds ratios, that if the 95% confidence interval of the odds ratio contains the value 1, there is no significant increase or decrease in the odds of developing the outcome based on the weight of that covariate. Now, an example will hopefully illustrate the nature of the plot. Five manuscripts were included in a **meta-analysis** of features of Huntington's Disease (HD). After careful elimination of manuscripts that characterized different cohorts of HD

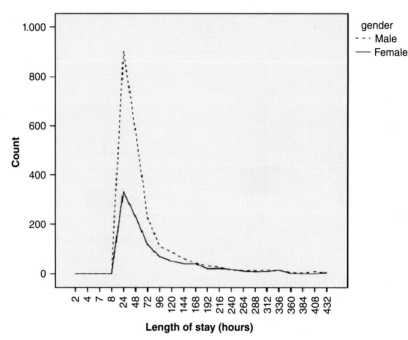

Figure 10.6 Line graph.

patients, five manuscripts made it through the rigorous selection process that is customary for meta-analyses.

See more on meta-analyses online.[39]

We noticed similarities in the findings between these five cohorts and wondered if being Caucasian added to the risk of bipolar depression in HD patients. So, each manuscript stated the odds ratios in their cohorts, and since I was doing the meta-analysis, I plotted the odds ratios and their 95% confidence intervals for all five cohorts onto one **forest plot** (Figure 10.7).

So, with the outcome having bipolar depression (absent = 0, present = 1) and the covariate being Caucasian (0 = no, 1 = yes), I see from the forest plot that two 95% confidence intervals of the odds ratios covered 1, which simply shows that being Caucasian did not increase the odds of developing bipolar depression.

10.8   Levey–Jennings Quality Control Chart

The **Levey–Jennings chart** is the most common **quality control (QC)** chart used in clinical laboratories to monitor external quality controls;

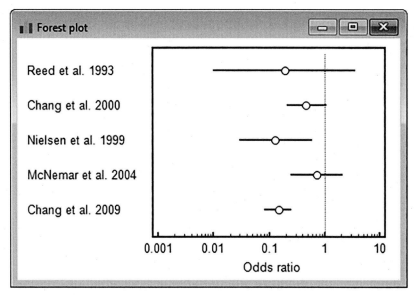

Figure 10.7 Forest plot.

more information can be obtained online.[40] It is a chart in which individual control measurements are plotted directly onto a control chart with limit lines drawn as the mean ± selected standard deviation (e.g., 2SD or 3SD). Time (days of a run) or runs are displayed on the x-axis and OD/CO values of the external control are plotted on the y-axis. Figure 10.8 shows a Levey–Jennings chart including the standard deviations around the mean.

By plotting data points (external control values) for each run, it is easy to interpret if changes are occurring. Ideally, the data points should distribute themselves around the mean value (above and below), because this is what determines a mean. Dramatic changes, or changes in direction or duration of changes in a direction, signal possible errors (random or systematic). Such changes are discussed below. Therefore, results on this type of control chart show individual data points as they occur and their relationship to the established mean, so that the sequence of results evolving over time can be readily visualized. Statistically, the results are followed so that situations where results signal a problem, or tend toward being out of control, are identified. Figures 10.9 and 10.10 show Levey–Jennings charts where shifts and trends have occurred, respectively (standard deviation values are not shown).

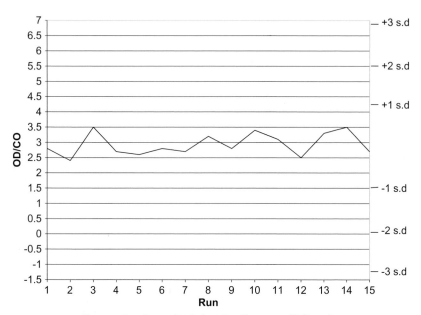

Levey–Jennings chart showing the mean (3.0) and standard deviations for 15 runs of an external control.

Figure 10.8 Levy–Jennings quality control chart.

10.8.1   Interpretation of QC Results

Each laboratory must determine the statistical methods and rules for establishing acceptability of external controls. For subsequent runs, it is expected that the external control values will fall on both sides of the mean with essentially equal frequency. An example of rules that could be applied is listed below.

Rules for Rejecting an External Control Value

- The external control results exceed two standard deviations from the mean.
- Or, the external controls exceed three standard deviations.
- Or, the external controls exceed two standard deviations on two consecutive days.

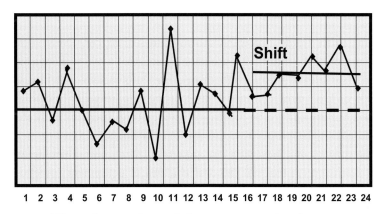

Time (e.g., day, date, run number)

Figure 10.9 Levy–Jennings chart demonstrating a shift in QC results.

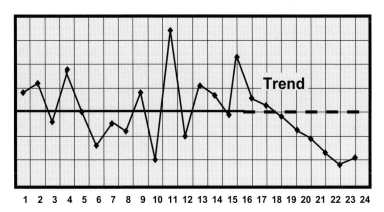

Time (e.g., day, date, run number)

Figure 10.10 Levy–Jennings chart demonstrating a trend in QC results.

- When it is expected that the values should be within two standard deviations 95% of the time, 5% of the time the values will be outside this range due to random error (not due to test kit or operator error).

Note that this is an example and the reader may need to seek the advice of regulatory agencies, if required.

10.8.2   Shifts and Trends

In general, **shifts** are defined when control values of six consecutive runs fall on one side of the mean. This usually indicates that a major change has occurred. Examples of situations that can cause shifts include switching to a new lot of kits (most common cause), using new reagents (including fresh wash buffer), changes in incubation temperatures (perhaps the water bath was not at the proper temperature or was not turned on), a new technologist (who may have different pipetting techniques), a contaminated or destroyed control sample, and changes of equipment (pipettes, plate washer, etc.). Shifts in the mean usually indicate that a systematic error has occurred.

Trends occur when six successive points become distributed in one general direction; that is, they are showing a gradual increase or decrease in values. This is usually the result of slowly changing parameters such as deterioration of reagents (conjugates are the most common cause, followed by changes in the control sample) or kit controls, or faltering equipment (e.g., a routinely used pipette is slowly losing its calibration).

It should be re-emphasized that when variation is identified through the use of the QC system, the entire test system should be reviewed to identify any causes of variation from the expected results. This will involve examining the entire testing process and assessing the integrity of each of its critical control parts. However, when a failure occurs, there is little that can be done beyond retesting all samples once the system is in control, so that inaccurate results are not released, and the system can be fixed.

Links to Online Tools

[39] https://www.meta-analysis.com/pages/why_do.php?cart
[40] www.westgard.com/lesson12.htm

Glossary

Analysis of variance (ANOVA): A comparison of two or more means and standard deviations for the purpose of examining differences between continuous measures of different groups.

Binary or dichotomous data: Non-continuous data that have just two options, i.e., yes/no, off/on, positive/negative.

Bivariate analysis: A procedure that compares one variable to another, or compares one variable between groups of the sample, e.g., comparison of height by weight or weight by gender.

Bonferroni correction: Lowering the threshold of significance to adjust for multiple comparisons.

Central Limit Theorem: Continuous draws of a measurement from all possible measurements, like weight measurements, that, with multiple sampling, will eventually take on a normal distribution (if the variable is inherently normally distributed).

Central tendency: A term used to describe the middle of a distribution of continuous data; the mean, median, or mode are types of central tendency measures.

Chi-square test 2×2 tables, aka contingency tables: A comparison of two binary variables that results in a comparison of proportions. It is a comparison of observed proportions minus expected proportions.

Coefficient of variation: The percentage of departure from the mean of a variable relative to the mean, which is calculated as the standard deviation divided by the mean of the distribution of the values.

Confidence intervals: Boundaries of the sample data distribution in which 90%, 95%, or 99% of data in the universe will reside, depending on where you set the boundaries, or how much error you are willing to accept. The lower the confidence intervals, the more error you will accept in how the data are truly distributed in the universe.

Continuous data: Quantitative data that begin at low values and extend to their natural upper boundaries or scale data ranging from zero to infinity, e.g., miles, weight, feet, height.

Cox proportional hazards model: A Kaplan–Meier life table where you can control for confounding covariables. It will generate a hazards ratio of developing the outcome (e.g., cancer death) given the effect of the covariable (e.g., cancer stage, age, or comorbidities).

Data management: The practice of handling the manner in which data are formatted, documented, verified, and validated.

Effect size: The size of the expected difference in measurements between two samples, or the strength of a correlation, or a proportion of a population.

Equivalence: Two sets of measurements are quantitatively equal within their 95% confidence intervals.

Fisher's exact test: When any of the cell entries in a chi-square table contain five or fewer observations, the P-value associated with Fisher's exact test is the appropriate value to report.

Frequency distributions: A list of all values in the data distribution and the number of instances of each value.

Geometric mean: A method used to find the central tendency, mean, and standard deviation data that reside in very different scales. For example, the mean of 1, 2, 1, 1, 490, 5660, and 10,000 would best be expressed as a geometric mean. Geometric means can also be used to find the central tendency of log-distributed data.

Hazards ratio: Usually generated in the analysis of time to events, the hazards ratio is relative to the effect of a covariable rather than the risk that the covariable imposes. If the hazards ratio is 2, a person with a particular trait (or covariate, like stage 4 cancer) will reach an endpoint twice as quickly as those with stage 3 cancer or less.

Hypotheses (alternate and null): A predetermined prediction about relationships between variables. The null hypothesis is the standard of no relationship, while the alternate hypothesis is your predetermined relationship. Such hypotheses are usually derived from the literature, or by experience or observation. Researchers may present primary and secondary hypotheses, where the primary is the main or most important hypothesis and the secondary is often exploratory in nature.

Interquartile range: Values found at the 25% and 75% points of the distribution.

Kaplan–Meier analysis: The most commonly used "time-to-event" analysis that accounts for censored events, due to loss to follow-up, or death before reaching the event of interest, e.g., time to death, remission-free survival.

Kappa statistic: A measure of agreement of a binary designation between two observers that takes into account the possibility that the agreement was caused by chance.

Kendall's tau: A correlation procedure that is made on paired (not independent), continuous measures.

Kurtosis: This describes the shape of your data distribution, whether all values are highly centered around the mean, or whether the values are more spread out towards the tails of the distribution.

Log_{10}-distributed data: Data distributions that follow a log_{10} scale, i.e., $1 \rightarrow 10 \rightarrow 100 \rightarrow 1000 \ldots$

Logistic regression: An analysis that examines the impact of covariates on the variance in the binary outcome variable. It generates an odds ratio of developing the binary outcome (y) given the presence or exposure of the covariate (x).

Log-rank test: Used to statistically compare survival "curves" of two or more groups.

Mean: Sum of all values divided by the number of values.

Median: The midpoint (50% cumulative frequency) between the lowest and highest value of the variable.

Meta-analysis: A comparison of methods and results of published clinical trials, or other types of studies, that are nearly identical in their sample selection, study treatments and placebos, and in similar environments. Rare diseases are difficult to study epidemiologically since it is difficult to gather data on more than a few cases per site. Thus, small studies are often mined from the literature base and compared to infer patterns within the disease across multiple studies; this type of comparison is called a meta-analysis.

Mode: The value occurring most frequently in the distribution.

Multiple comparisons: Making more than 20 statistical comparisons within groups or between groups of data.

Natural log: Data distributions that follow natural, incremental increases, i.e., $2 \rightarrow 4 \rightarrow 8 \rightarrow 16$, and so on. Incremental increases need not always be a doubling, but could be a tripling or more.

Non-continuous data: Ordinal data (strongly disagree = 0 to strongly agree = 5), binary data (yes = 1/no = 0), nominal data (1 = purple, 2 = pink, 3 = red...).

Non-inferiority: One effect of an agent is neither better nor worse than the effect of another agent.

Non-normally distributed continuous data: Data that are skewed to the right or to the left of center, so when plotted, their distributions lean to the right or to the left. Data that do not conform to a normal distribution.

Normally distributed continuous data: When plotted, normally distributed continuous data form a bell-shaped distribution where the mean is approximately equal to the median.

Odds ratios: This quantity expresses the likelihood that an outcome will occur as a result of an exposure(s).

One-sided vs. two-sided hypothesis testing: If one has the preconceived knowledge that an effect, such as the mean weight for Group A, will be heavier for men than for women, a one-tailed test is used since you expect the mean to be heavier rather than heavier or lighter. If you don't know which direction the effect will go, use a two-sided test.

Ordinal data: Non-continuous data that are ordered, i.e., strongly disagree = 0 to strongly agree = 5.

P-values: Represent the probability that comparisons between groups or variables are statistically different or correlated by chance alone. We usually accept significance at $P \leq 0.05$, or at more stringent levels, e.g., $P \leq 0.01$. For example, "patients in Group A were significantly heavier than patients in Group B, $P = 0.043$" means that the chance that this statistically significant finding happened by chance alone is ≤ 0.05, or $\leq 5\%$.

Paired T-test: A statistical method that compares paired measurements from the same individual; the means and standard deviations must be related. For example, weight before vs. after intervention.

Parametric vs. non-parametric analyses: A set of statistical tools used to evaluate normally vs. non-normally distributed data, respectively.

Pearson correlation: A statistical test that measures the degree of a relationship between two, normally distributed, continuous variables such as age or weight.

Power: The power is the probability that the test will reject a false designation of test inaccuracy, i.e., a false null finding. Power can either be calculated from the sample size and size of the effect, or power can be set in instances when you are calculating sample size.

Precision: Repeatability and reproducibility of a test or procedure.

Range: Lowest value to highest value of a variable.

Regression analysis (multivariate and multivariable analyses): Similar to a logistic regression but the outcome variable is a continuous variable, like weight or number of cells. A multivariable regression generates regression coefficients that explain the variance in a single outcome variable, while the multivariate regression explains the variance in two or more outcome variables.

Relative risk: The probability that an outcome will occur as a result of an exposure relative to the probability of an outcome occurring with non-exposure.

Repeatability: Otherwise known as **test–retest reliability**, and as a component of **precision**, repeatability is the measure of agreement of the same measurement taken on successive runs, under the same conditions, by the same technician, using the same equipment.

Reproducibility: As another component of **precision**, reproducibility is the ability of a test to produce the same results as another run when repeated by other technicians, in other conditions, and using other equipment.

ROC analysis: A non-statistical procedure used to find optimal cutoffs of continuous data for discriminating values into two groups, high and low. An example might be for a psychological test that tests for dyslexia, forming a final score that is a continuous variable. There is an optimal point along that numeric continuum where those above it have dyslexia and those scoring below that point do not have dyslexia.

Sample size: The number of patients or objects that will be necessary to determine the relationship of one variable to another, or a comparison between two or more groups, or one proportion of a population.

Sample vs. population: Sample is your randomly selected, representative collection of entities, while population is the universe that your sample represents.

Scatterplot: A graph showing the values of continuous measures on the x- and y-axes to show their linear relationship.

Skewness: Refers to the symmetry of the values around the mean of the distribution.

Spearman rank or Spearman's rho coefficient (independent observations): The non-parametric equivalent of a Pearson correlation but with non-normally distributed data.

Standard deviation: A measure of variation in your sample relative to the mean of your sample. A sum of the distances of each value to the mean of values.

Standard error: A measure of variation in the universe relative to the mean of the universe. It is also standard deviation/number of values.

Time-to-event data (life tables): A table that shows the kinetics of events occurring in a cohort or sample over time and calculates the median time to event for the cohort or cohorts. Each time an event occurs, like death, the cohort line drops vertically and then continues horizontally until the next event occurs.

T-test: A test that compares two independent means and standard deviations against each other; these means must be from two samples that are not related, such as boys and girls.

Type I error: This is the probability of rejecting a false positive when the false positive is true.

Type II error: This is the probability of accepting a false negative when the false negative is true (or a false null hypothesis).

Univariate analysis: An examination of one variable, such as mean, median, mode, etc.

Variable: A qualitative or quantitative unit that stratifies a population or group, or that measures a parameter, respectively. You may also see synonyms such as field, entry, value.

Wilcoxon rank sum test (aka Mann–Whitney *U*) of two independent samples: A way to compare non-normally distributed data of two independent samples.

Z-score: Z is a constant taken from a table of Z-scores; it represents the number of standard deviations from the mean.

Figure Credits

Figure 3.11	Courtesy of Zhiyong Johnny Zhang and Ke-Hai Yuan of WebPower.
Figure 3.12	Courtesy of Zhiyong Johnny Zhang and Ke-Hai Yuan of WebPower.
Figure 4.1	Created by the author.
Figure 4.2(a)	Created by the author.
Figure 4.2(b)	Created by the author.
Figure 4.3(a)	Created by the author.
Figure 4.3(b)	Created by the author.
Figure 4.3(c)	Created by the author.
Figure 4.4	Created by the author.
Figure 4.5	Created by the author.
Figure 4.6	Created by the author.
Figure 4.7	Courtesy of StatsKingdom.com
Figure 4.8	Courtesy of StatsKingdom.com
Figure 4.9	Courtesy of StatsKingdom.com
Figure 5.1(a)	Created by the author.
Figure 5.1(b)	Created by the author.
Figure 6.1	Courtesy of www.socscistatistics.com/tests/chisquare2/default2.aspx
Figure 6.2	Courtesy of www.socscistatistics.com/tests/chisquare2/default2.aspx
Figure 6.3	Courtesy of www.socscistatistics.com/tests/chisquare2/default2.aspx
Figure 6.4	Created by the author.
Figure 7.1	Courtesy of https://people.emich.edu/aross15/coursepack3419/logistic-javascript.html
Figure 7.2	Courtesy of https://people.emich.edu/aross15/coursepack3419/logistic-javascript.html
Figure 7.3(a)	Created by the author.
Figure 7.3(b)	Created by the author.
Figure 7.3(c)	Created by the author.
Figure 7.4	Created by the author.
Figure 8.1	Courtesy of the World Bank, licensed under CC BY-4.0 (https://datacatalog.worldbank.org/public-licenses#cc-by).
Figure 8.2	Courtesy of Zhiyong Johnny Zhang and Ke-Hai Yuan of WebPower.

Figure 8.3	Created by the author.
Figure 8.4	© 2015 Ahmed TA. Published in TA Ahmed (Ed.), *Basic Pharmacokinetic Concepts and Some Clinical Applications* under CC BY-3.0 license. Available at dx.doi.org/10.5772/61573
Figure 8.5	Pharmwiki (http://tmedweb.tulane.edu/pharmwiki/doku.php)
Figure 9.1	Adapted from Weuve Herbert LE, Weuve J, Scherr PA, Evans DA (2013) Alzheimer's Disease in the US (2010–2050) estimated using the 2010 census. *Neurology* 80(19): 1778–1783.
Figure 10.1	Created by the author.
Figure 10.2	Created by the author.
Figure 10.3	Created by the author.
Figure 10.4	Created by the author.
Figure 10.5	Created by the author.
Figure 10.6	Created by the author.
Figure 10.7	© 2020 MedCalc Software Ltd. Available at https://www.medcalc.org/manual/forestplot.php
Figure 10.8	Created by the author.
Figure 10.9	Created by the author.
Figure 10.10	Created by the author.

Index